Tobey Gross

DOPAMINE MACHINE

The Neuropsychological Cost of Escalating Social Approval

MINKOWSKI
Institute Press

Dr. Tobey Gross
Professor of Educational Science
www.tobeygross.de

ISBN: 978-1-998902-47-7 (softcover)
ISBN: 978-1-998902-48-4 (ebook)

Minkowski Institute Press
Montreal, Quebec, Canada
https://minkowskiinstitute.com/mip/

For information on all Minkowski Institute Press publications
visit our website at https://minkowskiinstitute.com/mip/books/

To Joline and Christopher

May your love always grow and bloom as prosperous as the mold would on the leftover sandwiches in my school bag that I forgot to dispose on the last day of school before the summer holidays each year, much to the ire of my mother.

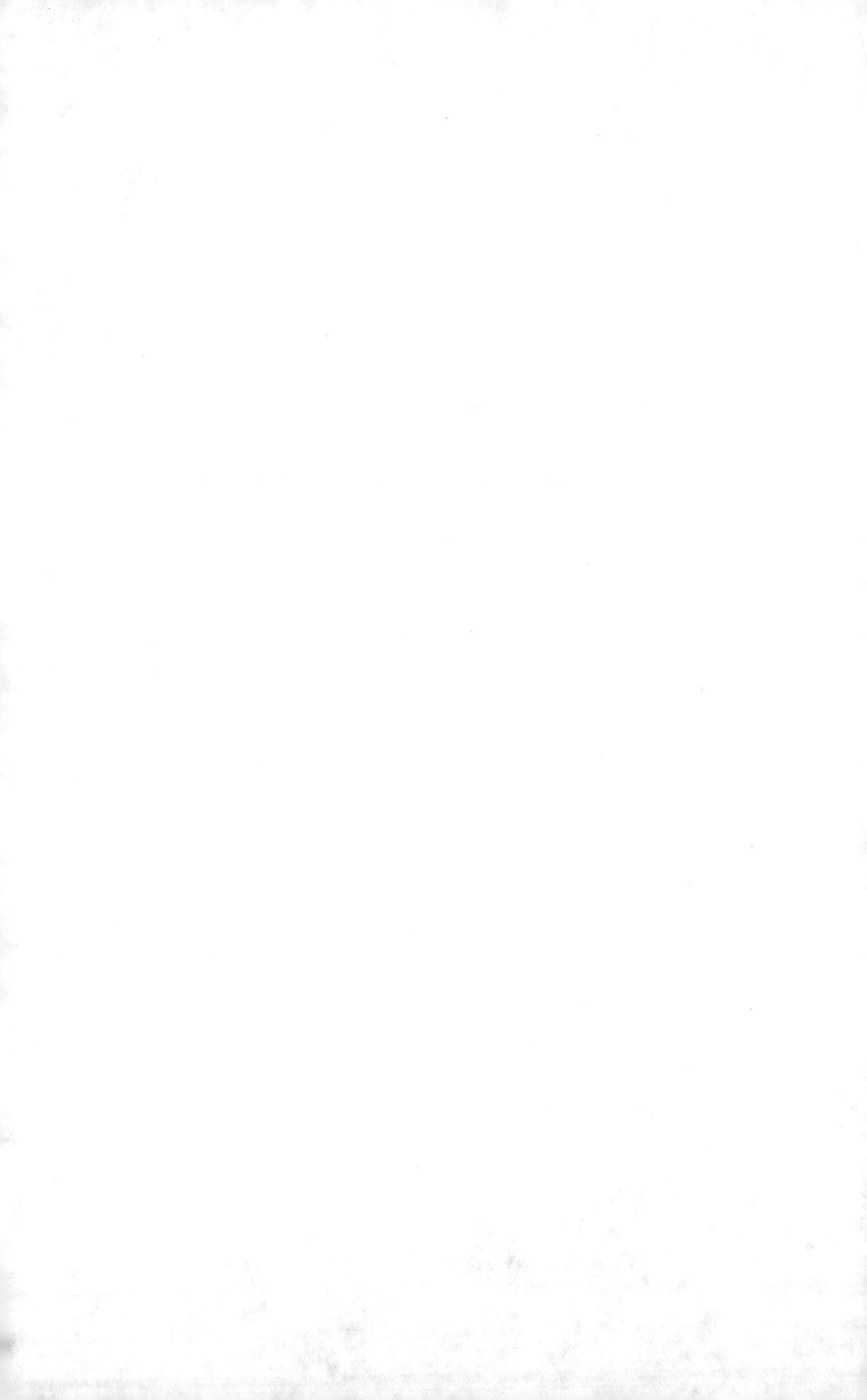

CONTENTS

iv

1 INTRODUCTION: PURPOSE OF THIS WORK

In a time where technology promises unprecedented connectivity, individuals find themselves paradoxically isolated, locked in a relentless cycle of comparison and validation. Digital personas, algorithm-driven feedback loops and superficial representation of made-up personas expose fundamental tension between humanity's ancient social instincts and the rapidly evolving digital architecture of society. This work aims to venture into the depths of these tensions and to explain the collision between ancestral behavioral frameworks and contemporary digital life. This clash unveils our need for social validation but has also created a new form of social currency that fundamentally drives modern human behavior, often to harmful extremes.

The promise of digital networks was to democratize global connectivity, enabling individuals to share their lives and broadcast their identities with a global audience. Yet beneath this veneer of accessibility lies a potent mechanism of psychological manipulation, as social media platforms capitalize on neurobiological patterns that we can not simply switch off. Variable reinforcement schedules, embedded in seemingly harmless social interactions, transform these platforms into powerful triggers of dopamine-driven behavior. The paradox in this integration of behavioral science into technology is the authentic search of individuals for connection to society while eventually finding themselves more isolated and excluded, through amplification of inadequacy and innate inferiority.

This analysis aims to present a unified and holistic perspective on the forces at play. It delves beyond the ascent of digital platforms and integrates neuroscientific aspects and foundational psychological theories in modern social structures, media and behavioral insights, while sharing experience in the work with individuals who are trying to exit the vicious cycles composed of reward-craving behavioral patterns. It unveils how the neurobiological makeup is unable to adapt to the ever accelerating changes in society and how our brain chemicals send us deeper into the trap.

At the cost of what makes us sustainably happy, we have become heavily reliant on short-term phasic dopamine, which can hinder the balance of neurotransmitters in our brains, creating a lasting source of dissatisfaction.

We aim to explain each component in depth, before synthesizing the different perspectives from a larger lens. It will become obvious how we engage in a massive trade-off, where dopamine becomes our main objective in modern life, through societal structures that foster these behavioral patterns. We will learn how difficult it is to put an end to this loop because our brains physically and chemically adapt over time. At the end, shared experiences will give insights into strategies that can be applied in the work with individuals seeking support.

1.1 The historical context of social validation

In the earliest stages of human development, belonging to a community was crucial for survival. A larger group conferred strength, significantly decreasing the risk of falling prey to predators. In contrast, individuals living alone faced considerable dangers from the environment. Being part of a larger community provided not only protection from natural threats but also access to vital resources such as food. The collective defense of both individuals and shared resources benefited all members of the group. Given the myriad and unpredictable threats present in the wild, shared vigilance and threat detection became invaluable assets for the community. From these tribal origins, humans recognized that forming groups was essential for survival and facilitated stable access to necessary natural resources. The formation of strong relationships emerged as a fundamental pillar of group stability and support for each individual.

In challenging environments, mutual aid and collaborative problem-solving became integral to group dynamics. Collective efforts in activities such as hunting, building shelter, sharing knowledge, and providing reciprocal assistance allowed for the pooling of skills and strengths for the common good. Long-term cohesion within groups depended on trust-building, as establishing reliability was critical for sustainable functioning and benefiting all members. Consequently, exclusion from a group posed a severe risk to an individual; being barred from the group's resources, shelter, and assistance heightened exposure to dangers in the wild, which individuals could withstand only for a limited time. Vulnerability would be significantly amplified, and available countermeasures were minimal. The emotional impact of exclusion from a tribal community would have been considerable.

Given the harsh and unforgiving environments of the time, the limited resources available for selfsustenance created strong incentives for conformity within groups and discouraged behaviors that could lead to exclusion. In line with the principle of survival of the fittest, tribal individuals developed traits that enhanced their ability to thrive within social structures. The process of natural selection favored those traits in social individuals, as such traits increased their chances of reproduction and survival across generations. Consequently, behaviors promoting group living and cooperation became genetically favored over time. This included innate social instincts that evolved to facilitate collaboration for both individual and group benefit. Shaped by environmental pressures, this adaptation of social behavior represents a form of "behavioral evolution," laying the groundwork for flexible responses to social environments and an inherent understanding of the importance of group cohesion and conformity.

As these social instincts solidified, they became the bedrock upon which early societies were built. The most fundamental of these social units were the clan and tribal systems, where kinship bonds played a crucial role. Family-based groups, tied by blood relations, formed the core units of early social structures. These bonds ensured that individuals were deeply connected through shared ancestry, creating strong social ties that were vital for survival and mutual support. Systemic structures remained as they had been, with shared access to resources and skills necessary for group survival, mutual aid and benefit. Resources were shared among the clan and distributed among its members, sheltered from foreign threats. A form of communal ownership emerged, with group consensus being the asset that sustained and secured group living. Leaders often emerged naturally, based on their specific superiority over other group members.

What had begun in small tribal communities as a system of inner cohesion and guarded groups, would now begin to reproduce at a larger scale, when groups formed alliances and inter-group relations would form over time. Befriended groups would share intelligence and resources, conflicts with other groups would emerge, interactions between clans would determine their status toward one another. In those solidified social groups, with authority figures with decision-making power, a sense of social stratification assigned rank and status to individual group members, often based on their skills, gender and natural strength. Here, the first division of labor would assign individuals their clearly determined role within the group, assigning them an individual sense of identity. While control over resources and decisions were maintained by those in higher status, each member of a group had a defined role to fulfill and would develop an identity based on their systemic role in the greater group dynamics.

With the emergence of group rituals, ceremonial practices, rites of passage etc., group cohesion was reinforced, which would especially be valuable for the sense of belonging and at the same time, further define the shared beliefs, moral codes and group values, that can be understood as the guidelines for desired individual behavior. In that regard, community judgment evolved, and with it the first sense of social standing, within a more complex system of societal approval and disapproval. The shared traditions and social norms formed collective identity, that was slowly becoming more than a survival-securing "pack"-sense, because it would build on many more values over time, like shared ancestry, community identity in the form of cultural practice and customs that bound the group as a community. Group loyalty was getting more symbolic and had an emotional aspect to it, rather than just ensuring resource access and shelter from external threats. As a strong allegiance to the group, often represented by symbols or objects, represented loyalty and belonging, an understanding of prioritization emerged, valuing group loyalty higher than individual needs.

As societies grew more complex, so too did the frameworks that governed social behavior. This gave rise to the development of social norms, which became essential in regulating the interactions within these burgeoning communities. The emergence of cultural norms provided a set of established behaviors and customs that were passed down through generations. These norms served as the unwritten rules of society, guiding acceptable behavior and ensuring that individuals adhered to the shared values that unified the group. The changes in norms were defined by societal needs, with individuals in the group adapting. The emergence of religion and traditions provided moral frameworks, that fostered desired behavior, and likewise reinforced cultural values in order to maintain social cohesion. Sustaining these practices and passing them on to following generations linked present to ancestral ways.

Social reinforcement functioned to a large extent through reward and punishment, with groups gradually developing penalty systems for deviating behavior and likewise, rewarding conformity by social status. Maintenance of group harmony could, given the evolution of more complex societal dynamics and growing communities, only be achieved through law and order; formalized rules were being set. This led to collective reinforcement of predefined rules, with behavioral conditioning through sanctioning undesired and deviant behavior, while rewarding participation and obeyance.

These new systems could be perceived as the first social pressure, by the prevalent strong encouragement of conform behavior. Individual expression and forming an individual identity had to function within the boundaries of society, which could be an act of balancing individual needs with greater expectations from the group. Tension between roles was consequently an inherent nature of individuality vs. conformity.

1.2 Objective: A Comprehensive Synthesis of and Theory on Modern Social Validation Issues

Evaluating the origins of social validation, is has been vital for human survival through securement of crucial resources and individual protection against harsh environmental threats, benefiting each individual member of the group. Strong social bonds were perceived as a necessity to enhance chances of survival and also ensure reproduction, hence over time, natural selection would genetically favor socially approved behavior in individuals. Consequently, fostering well-being, our brains have evolved to be particularly responsive to social feedback, with the evolutionary development of neurochemical responses like dopamine release. This neurochemical reinforcement of social acceptance was an essential feature for maintaining group cohesion over thousands of years and potentially secured human survival until the present day.

However, in today's society, the innate need for social validation has intensified, often exceeding the evolutionary capacities. Modern individuals receive social feedback not only in vastly different forms than our ancestors, but also from a wide array of sources. While originally, social acceptance and validation was only critical from immediate circles, and only provided by them, in today's society, individuals receive feedback from large communities, workplaces, social platforms, mass media and so on. In comparison, this vastly expanded landscape of social interaction presents challenges that can overwhelm our natural feedback mechanisms. One could say, that the innate mechanisms for the adaptation to social feedback was just not designed for the array of social feedback we permanently receive. Contemporary environments are inundated with a continuous stream of input, that shapes our perceptions of beauty, self-worth, success. Advertisements, social media, television and various other forms of consumed media constantly present idealized images and narratives about how life "should be". This consistent exposure can, arguably, increase feelings of inferiority – a concept extensively discussed by Alfred Adler, who suggested, that humans are inherently motivated by feelings of inferiority and the drive to overcome them. This particular aspect of human behavior will play a crucial role in later elaborations.

Today's relentless presentations of perfect or near-perfect representations of others, whether through advertising or social media, induces a state of perpetual upward comparison in consumers. Interestingly, even portrayals of "flawed" or "ordinary" individuals are often idealized, depicting them as navigating life's challenges effortlessly. This never-ending stream of idealized imagery exacerbates the deeply entrenched feelings of inadequacy. That is where the bridge is: Perpetuated feelings of inadequacy, reinforced through permanent exposure to people better than ourselves, amplify the automation in upward comparison and fuel the innate inferiority perceptions, having individuals longing for ever more social validation to offset their emotional imbalances.

These dynamics create a highly potent interplay of craving, anxiety and perceived inferiority, to life, if you will. Craving for the soothing effect of validation is deeply rooted in our brains' neurochemical makeup; dopamine-driven anticipation of social rewards like recognition, praise, and approval in everyday interactions with other human beings. Each instance of social approval results in dopamine release, reinforcing the behavior of seeking further approval. How these dynamics function exactly, will be explained. However, the ongoing exposure to ever-idealized standards is also an excellent trigger for feelings of inadequacy and social anxiety: the fear of not meeting social standards, societal expectations and the potential for (perceived) rejection. As mentioned earlier, exposure to large circles of potential feedback increases the perceived rejection from society at large, likewise. The leveraged effect of receiving feedback from large circles through modern channels works in both positive and negative ways.

Again, this fear of inadequacy is deeply rooted in our evolutionary history, where social rejection and exclusion from the community could pose no less than an existential threat to an individual. In contemporary contexts, the anxiety stemming from failure to meet societal ideals, compounded by relentless comparisons, can lead to heightened stress and a perpetually fueled search for validation.

Over time, the vast mismatch between our evolutionary psychological makeup and modern social dynamics can contribute to emotional instability, particularly resulting in amplitudinal, volatile frequency cycles, sometimes vaguely reminiscent of bipolarity. Dopamine-induced "highs" from social validation are followed by "low" periods when feedback is absent or (perceived) negative. While high on dopamine, individuals feel motivated and experience pleasure, the fading effect leaves them with feelings of emptiness, worthlessness and solitude.

On a neurochemical level, it is arguable, whether the behavior, that gradually shifts to frequently seeking dopamine rushes, has a disruptive nature to the delicate balance of neurochemicals in our brain: specifically the balance between dopamine, which is the neurotransmitter responsible for plea-sure and motivation, and serotonin, which regulates mood and is more associated with general emotional stability and well-being. It is an interesting question, if the frequent over-stimulation and exposure to external stimuli has long-term effects on the serotonin balance, since we know, that those two neurotransmitters interact in frequent ways. As the brain works to manage the overwhelming influx of social feedback and permanent comparison, inducing high rushes and inferio-rity-induced lows, imbalances might be responsible for anxi-ety, mood swings and also depressive characteristics.

Further complications in these dynamics can be attributed to the well-established fact, that modern social validation, of-ten in digital form, resemble so-called variable reinforcement patterns, or variably-scheduled reinforcement, as they were first identified by B. F. Skinner in the first half of the 20th century. It could be evidenced, that a rather unpredictable nature in reinforcement, i. e. not knowing about the reward triggering a neurochemical response, would significantly am-plify compulsive behavior, resembling addiction. The more unpredictable a reward is, the more compulsively an individ-ual will "pull the lever". These findings in early behavioral science function like a blueprint for modern social validation patterns, often trapping an individual's brain in a cycle of seeking validation, while at the same time fearing rejection and feeling inferior. All these dynamics might lead to persis-tent mental health challenges over time, because our brains are not evolutionarily designed for these cycles.

The objective of this work is bridging and synthesizing evolutionary psychology, neurochemical processes and mod-ern social dynamics to offer an original framework on how social validation functions in contemporary society and what the effects of persistent upward comparisons, expansive so-cial feedback and dopamine-driven behavioral patterns are. Under the lens of biological predispositions and in a broader context of digital media and contemporary behavioral science, this work aims to investigate emotional imbalances and dysfunctions as a potential consequence of modern social dynamics, integrating Adler's concept of inferiority.

2 EVOLUTIONARY FOUNDATIONS OF SOCIAL VALIDATION

2.1 Evolutionary Psychology: Understanding Human Behavior Through Ancestry

While in tribal ages, being alone was a high risk, because isolation meant a rather small chance of survival (Marlowe, 2005), individuals were early to learn, that social bonds were beneficial for increased chances to stay alive. The dangers that very early humans faced were numerous and harsh. For instance, even a minor injury could develop to become a major infection, for which no medical treatment was available, and might potentially lead to death (Gamble, 1999). Limited healing and practically zero immunity caused high mortality rates in early human individuals, from virtually any sort of disease (Aiello & Wheeler, 1995). Apart from that, they were exposed to numerous threats and dangers, that would constantly pose significants risks of death (Boyd & Silk, 2018); be it large carnivores that were ready to attack any moment, extremely harsh climates or natural disasters, scarcity in resources, food and water, or peer violence for whatever reason (Boehm, 1999; Kaplan et al., 2000; Foley, 2002; Hart & Sussman, 2005).

Bowlby (1969), Lovejoy (1981), Kelly (1995) and Sikora et al. (2017) describe the first forms of social bonding as a survival imperative; group defense and the avoidance of and protection against predators were a mandatory element of securing prolonged survival. Safety in numbers was practically the only way to cope with the various existential threats at the time (Pearce & Moutsiou, 2014). Mutual support extended beyond protection of the tribe, since reproduction, embedded in genetics, would necessarily demand pairing and cooperative breeding and group-based child rearing would also increase survival rates (Hrdy, 2009; Alvard, 2009). Hamilton (1964) describes early kinship in family-ties, that stayed together closely. Shared genes would fasten social bonds. Tasks that were necessary to maintain the tribe were executed cooperatively, through sharing of resources and cooperation in hunting (Isaac, 1978; Lee & DeVore, 1968). Clutton-Brock (1974) particularly describes the strategic locations of first communal living in tribes, specifically for the shared use of water, while Lee & DeVore (1968) found cooperative gathering of food, sharing of meat as an important natural resource and the reduced risk through cooperation in hunting and gathering as important factors of early communal benefits. Mutual support extended beyond hunting and gathering, since sickness and injuries were frequent and would require community care in order to maintain strength for the tribe as a whole (Gurven & Hill, 2009).

The requirements life demanded from early humans thus meant that life without a community would practically be impossible, which is why the tribal age can be seen as the origin of social life in humans. Living in communities can only function through cohesion, which includes a certain degree of set rules, that each member of the group must obey. Shared interests and needs and mutual aid, together with the avoidance of the manifold dangers would set an imperative for an individual to care for the maintenance of the tribe as well as for their own. That is, early social structures evolved, which included the differentiation of roles and rudimentary hierarchies within tribes (Boehm, 2012). While language and communication was rudimentary as well, gesture-based language patterns would be sufficient for the amount of communication needed (Tomasello, 2008). Basic social roles in early tribes were tightly affiliated with the essential tasks and were not yet meant to form a degree of identity, but were rather survival-driven, which is an important note at this point (Boehm, 1999); role differentiation was merely practical, often gender-based, in a hunter vs. gatherer schematic system and division of labor (Dunbar, 1993). It is an important part of understanding the formation process, because these social roles differ largely from those, that we know in modern times – in early tribes, the assignment of roles was not driven by self-actualization, but rather skill-based and survival-driven, enhancing the maximum of each individual's capabilities in order to secure maintenance of the tribe community (Woodburn, 1982). However, even then, leadership in the hierarchies evolved from experience, skills and wisdom, and thus belonged to the strongest, eldest and most capable. The eldest had the best knowledge of the environment, while hunting success displayed particularly well-developed skill sets and raw strength, which was an important asset for dominance and survival – the roles were achieved (Wiessner, 2002; Kelly, 1995; Lee & Daly, 1999; Woodburn, 1982; Dunbar, 1993; Sahlins, 1972). Furthermore, the social space was finite, with only the closest peers around, which limited the scope of recognition to a very small circle (Foley & Lee, 1989).

In summary, social acceptance of peers, as in its early form, was a survival-ensuring component of human life, and social standing was derived from individual capabilities. As survival was deeply intertwined with social bonds and group cohesion, and isolation was life-threatening, social approval was essential because it would ensure protection, food and shared resources. While roles in the tribe were based on practical skills and caregiving, social standing was only determined by the individual's capabilities of contributing to the tribe's survival. Social roles would solely have a functional meaning, since there was no broader societal validation. At the time, there was little room for self-expression, sense of identity or self, because one's worth was defined by their role in the tribe. However, this evolutionary foundation laid the groundwork for the more complex validation forms that would emerge in later societies.

The gradual expansion of human communities brought about new dimensions of societal complexity and with them, social roles began to diversify. As individuals started to be recognized for more than only their contribution to the community's immediate needs, social validation would become more intertwined with one's own sense of identity, which gradually led to a more nuanced understanding of an individual's role in the broader societal framework.

2.2 The Transition from Tribes to More Complex Societies

According to Simmel (1971), roles in society evolved along with societal complexity, factoring in the emergence of social norms and moral codes. As social circles and structures broadened, the development of an own sense of self and an identification process gradually launched in individuals; the identity formation was being linked to the perceived social structures (Turner, 1991).

A key element in the development of identity as we think about it these days was the emergence of language beyond rudimentary sounds and gestures. Language, according to Tomasello (2014) and Dunbar (1996), was the most important factor in the sense of self, because communication led to reflection and the first tangible development of the idea of a self. This process could be described as a cognitive expansion. As individuals began recognizing thoughts, intentions and feelings of others, it led to deeper forms of reflection on their own minds and personal identities (Humphrey, 1976). What emerged, were first groundstones for the Theory of Mind, that describes an individual's ability to reflect beyond their own thoughts and intentions, as well as beliefs, feelings and potential limitations, and become aware, that others may or may not share these, including the potential contrast in existing knowledge or experience, leading to much more nuanced interaction based on the acknowledgement of these dichotomies (Premack & Woodruff, 1978; Gross, 2023). Based on archeological evidence, Mithen (1996) describes the beginnings of a more complex sense of self through personal expression outside of the tribe role, which can be seen in rituals and the emergence of symbolic thinking, evident in early cave paintings.

What we observe in these crucial societal shifts is the fact, that survival became significantly easier for each individual over time, as communities stabilized and transitioned to agriculture; the mere gain of time to reflect and recognize own thoughts and feelings was based on the gradual fade of a constant alertness for potentially life-threatening dangers that would lurk virtually everywhere, at any time. Understandably, self-expression and reflection of thoughts and attitudes comes only second to not being eaten by a predator while picking berries. The growing stability in daily lives allowed for more space to develop personal identities beyond tribal roles, along with emergence of personal goals and moral responsibilities, shifting to individuals seeing themselves as independent beings with values and identity (McAdams, 1993; Renfrew, 2007; Taylor, 1989). The moral codes of society became more complex and nuanced, which had necessary effects on how individuals perceived their own status in the social system; while violations of social norms led to loss of status and privileges, an honor code developed, that would link an individual's personal behavior to expectations from broadening social cricles (Fukuyama, 2011).

Respect was gained through leadership, which included wisdom and capability, but also fairness, ethical conduct and justice, in line what was perceived as beneficial for society as a whole. As social groups grew larger, greater cooperation was required to maintain cohesion, so society would not fall apart. Social reputation served as an important factor of control, because it ensured conformity with social norms (Henrich & Gil-White, 2011; Flannery & Marcus, 2012). Honor, thus, became more central to an individual's self-perception and gradually replaced survival as a key motivation for social behavior (McAdams, 1993).

At this point, we may conclude, that the public image of an individual first began to matter, because consequently, society in its deepening and widening structures formed first images of idealized behavior with certain forms of reward and punishment upon the degree of conformity. This is confirmed by Richerson & Boyd (2005), who found that norms and group expectations shaped individual actions. Early societies relied on feedback for the regulation of individual behavior, which is ultimately another essential part of human evolution overall, besides genetic makeup. Interestingly, Johnson & Earle (2000) were able to find, that the degree of hierarchy within a society would have significant implications for the influence of social feedback on individual behavior. Likewise, status was tightly linked to the adherence in group norms. According to Barkow (1989), those in power used classic reward-punishment methods to shape desired behavior, known from conditioning techniques that will be discussed later on. Social rewards like status and praise were granted for desired behavior, while shame and exclusion were the consequence of anti-social actions. Individuals would internalize those structures early on.

Arguably, the internalization of these social regulating mechanisms quickly found their way into the upbringing of offspring, so it is not surprising, that genetic evolution and social evolution became intertwined, aligning with what Richerson & Boyd argued. The caretaking aspect of bringing up offspring had to include social aspects to ensure successful reproduction in the future. At that time, being social had already been internalized from tribal age, because individuals would learn early, that group cohesion ensured survival. The argumentation however remained, because exclusion from society, however small or large, would eventually mean no reproduction and overall, harm. It is crucial to understand, that while social systems and with them, individuals, grew more complex, the internal links had not changed much: being social meant benefit, not being social would not end well. Therefore, even though society had become more than a meaningful edge in chances of survival, the biological aspect of belonging was still as important as it had ever been, only expressed in more nuanced ways and through more complex feedback.

In line with the individual self-perception, hierarchy in social systems had significant influence on early forms of self-worth, not much different than in modern times. Lower status could diminish the self-concept while higher status led to an increase in self-worth; hierarchical settings, that determined one's place in the societal ranking had direct influence on the concept of personal identity (Turner, 1985).

2.3 Collective vs. Personal Identity and Community-Driven vs. Self-Driven Motivations for Validation

As has been described, in early societies, collective identity often took precedence over individual identity, since fulfilling responsibilities and expectation set by the collective would outweigh personal expression by much. This dynamic can be seen across various dimensions of social organization. Identities were closely intertwined with the roles assigned to individuals, mainly depending on age, status, and notably, gender. According to Knauft (1991), personal identity for men and women was based on the roles assigned to the gender. Collectively assigned, gender-based roles were rigid and left little room for exploration of personal identity outside of the realm of the own assigned circle.

However, as societies grew, personal achievements and the development of own awareness became more prevalent, status mattered. Personal identity and collective identity melted together more, which left more space for the pursuit of personal goals alongside collective responsibilities (McAdams, 1993).

The tension between collective needs and personal desires has been outlined in Thomas Hobbes's (1651) *Leviathan*, where he mentions the so-called *social contract*: Hobbes describes human nature as selfish in the way that humans are inherently wired to act in their own best interest, which leads to a state of constant conflict. To avoid the necessary conflict arising from chaos, individuals are willing to surrender some of their original freedom in exchange for security and order, which in turn forms a society. The dynamic Hobbes describes is a well-researched inner conflict of personal and collective identity, where collective needs are rooted in the need for the degree of social stability that each individual benefits from. This requires each individual to curb their personal desires for the greater good and strike a balance – the social contract. It is necessary, according to Hobbes, because in a state of ungoverned individual chaos, the fulfillment of personal desires becomes virtually impossible, which in turn makes for each individual's willingness to sacrifice total freedom for the common good, as well as their own.

As Hobbes concluded, the inner tension of the indivdual self vs. the collective was manifested in the expectations individuals had to meet. Navigating this balance became more complicated the more sophisticated societies became. One of the foundational thinkers in sociology, Emile Durkheim, describes simpler societies in what he terms *Mechanical Solidarity*, where communities are bound together by beliefs and values, and collective identity has much more weight than individual identity, enforced through social collective norms. The strong sense of collective belonging is mainly based on sharing common experiences and performing simple, similar tasks. In this form of society, the own sense of self is directly derived from an individual's standing and role within the collective. Throughout the evolution of societies, Durkheim describes his term *Organic Solidarity*, which means moving away from uniformity by the growing performance of more specialized tasks, with a growing interdependence. This allows more space for the exploration of the self and deriving more personal identity from one's own uniqueness. Despite more personal freedom of expression, cohesion within the collective remains an essential part of social structure, because with more interdependence, reliability and cooperation became even more important. However, Durkheim sees the growing complexity in societal systems as the main reason for the general decrease in shared identity.

As mentioned, since the balance between personal desire and collective need would not always be easy to find, and uncontrolled deviation might lead to imbalances in society, the collective needed governance. As labor was divised and leadership emerged, it required suppressing personal desires to ensure collective harmony. While individuals became more capable of discerning between the two, in a dual recognition of own needs and those of the community or other individuals, their mediation had to fit into a legal framework: laws and norms emerged, early states formed (Fried, 1967; Whiten & Byrne, 1997; Flannery, 1972; Johnson & Earle, 1987). On the other hand, Kohlberg (1981) describes a moral evolution in individuals, with the development of an own moral agency as one of the cornerstones of a greater personal identity, but in the constraints of collective needs. Lastly, religious structures in organized religion solidified group identity and belonging on an individual basis, because religious cults and rituals offered the individual the opportunity to express themselves within their hierarchies (Bellah, 2011).

Since religion consisted of collective activities, it was suitable to reinforce group cohesion and form stronger collective identification through shared beliefs (Durkheim, 1912); the so-called *common spiritual banner* provided a strong sense of belonging, since religious rituals required group participation, where personal identities were submerged under collective experience. However, religion provided room for personal development and individual standing in society, because it functioned through strong hierarchical order, where priests and shamans had their societal roles with an affiliated status (Lévi-Strauss, 1962; Turner, 1969; Eliade, 1958; Turchin, 2015). In later stages, state-endorsed religion provided new opportunities to establish a dual identification of the individual, shaped by loyalty to the state and also to the religious community (Assmann, 1997).

3 THE EVOLUTIONARY MISMATCH: MODERN SOCIETY VS. ANCESTRAL ENVIRONMENT

While early human societies operated in small and tight-knit groups, that were based on survival and proximity, over time, human interaction expanded further and further beyond immediate circles. The meaning and sophistication of own identification processes expanded with it, so that dynamics in social validation shifted towards wider social networks and other means of personality development than contribution to the tribe's survival and maintenance. The development of communication allowed for an exponential growth in social circles, from local to regional and eventually global communities.

In early tribal settings, social status had little meaning for the development of personal identities, especially because tasks were similar and repetitive and social roles were pragmatic, unreflected, not self-expressive and only tied to labor. It was only through diversification of society over time, that a conscious self would expand beyond survival tasks and introduce more nuanced layers of social approval and validation, in which individuals would find deeper meaning for themselves.

Through ever-growing societies and exposure, individuals are nowadays judged against global standards, presented with an ever-growing array of cultural expectations and unbelievably sophisticated degrees of self-expression on a global stage.

Since social validation has entirely shifted from being a survival imperative to sophisticated expressions of the self with no meaning for surviving, the complexity of social dynamics can easily become overwhelming, with the rising pressures of more and more defined societal standards from success over beauty to behavior, from skills to fame over materialistic ideals and status symbols. The following chapter will analyze these shifts in depth – the *mismatch* between evolutionary makeup and the exponential expansion of social validation; what does it do to our brains? And if humans have internalized the necessity of being social in their genetic code, did we likewise develop to handle modern means and arrays of social approval? Or did validation scales grow much larger than we did?

3.1 The Expansion of Social Networks: From Tribal Closeness to Global Communities

One of the most important shifts in social validation was the introduction of currency, which meant a significant move to wealth and trade. Social approval could be directly linked to economic success and was displayed visually (Smith, 2005, originally published in 1776). Currency allowed for more abstract and quantifiable measurements of worth, which replaced traditional status markers and introduced new social hierarchies (Davies, 1996). Indicators of wealth became much more external, while individuals focused on material success, contrasting pre-existing status hierarchies that had no affiliation to material acumen. Smith (1776) describes the shift in personal autonomy, since status could be achieved outside of traditional social structures (i. e. birthright or religion). As individual wealth became a primary measure of identity, social validation would become part of a sense for competition, where previously cultural or religious practices fostered collective identity. However, it would raise ambitions to participate in trade, while on the other hand, it certainly introduced novel forms of anxiety – no more focused on surviving and not being excluded from the tribe, but missing out on status markers. According to Graeber (2011), this shift also meant a significant shift in individual psyche, since the focal points in life drastically changed.

The introduction of money as the main metric of success has been subject of scholarly research from early on; Thorstein Veblen (1899) presented interesting theories on the socio-psychological effects. In his popular concept of *conspicuous consumption*, he refers to the habit of spending money on goods, that are unnecessary and particularly meant to display material wealth, in order to convince others of one's own economic power and gain social validation as a consequence. Veblen expanded on the concept and introduced his idea of *conspicuous leisure*, which describes an engagement in specific leisure activities, that are meant to signal to the outside, that the individual performing those activities does not need to work. The prominent display of wealth, according to Veblen's logic, created psychological dynamics that were specifically targeted to gain social approval through the prominent display of wealth.

As described before, Veblen observed early, that individuals developed the habit to compare themselves to others, to determine their own social status. Interestingly, this concept blends into the ideas of Alfred Adler, which will be adopted into this work at a later point. Likewise, it confirms the shift to more external status markers. With the shift in individual perception and awareness of others' externally displayed status, the internalization of own status could mean individual suffering: Veblen describes a cycle of competition for social validation, with the need to outdo others in consuming more and displaying even greater wealth. With the strong shift of social status to the outside, necessarily, intrinsic self-worth and traditional sense of status and self would decrease in importance. Self-esteem would gradually be linked to what, or how much, an individual could showcase. Lastly, Veblen observed, that particularly wasteful behavior was perceived as wealthy; thus, psychological validation was no more linked to productivity or communal contribution. The display of the ability to waste resources demonstrated economic – and thus *societal* – superiority.

Graeber (2011) sees social power dynamics especially in the alienation from labor. He describes, how the shift and formalization of monetary systems meant a psychological detachment from the actual work for communal benefit, towards work for wages. According to his findings, this means the control of wealth went along with social supremacy, which altered the individual psyche. The working individual cultivated a personal interest in wealth accumulation for power and validation, instead of communal benefit and survival of the group. However, the introduction of lending systems and debt brought forth the connection between morals, emotion and economy, fostering a notion of moral guilt in individuals with financial obligations. Being in debt was seen as failure or even morally wrong, which would affect self-esteem and identity to a high degree. With all these developments, social relationships became monetized; communal bonds eroded and shifted selfworth away from personal qualities, tying it closer to economic transactions – with profound implications for individual psychology.

Another important cornerstone was marked by the era of industrialization, where the importance of money grew further, along with skill and innovation spirit. When work shifted from agrarian to industrial, capital, entrepreneurship and investment became essential factors for the rise of the middle class. Social validation and wealth were no more only for the aristocracy; middle class found their primary identity in their professions, alongside the money that they provided for their immediate family. Also, education became an important factor for the later opportunities to belong and secure belonging. Personal success became tied to economic mobility (Polanyi, 1944; Thompson, 1963).

However, the rise of the middle class brought new competition into the now widening access to wealth and education and the accumulation of monetary assets. What followed was the need for approval in more anonymous and much wider social circles: the classic status symbol was born. According to Sennett (1977), McKendrick et al. (1982) and Hobsbawm (1968), important symbols were fashion, housing and public visibility. Veblen (1899) sees the ability to acquire mass-produced goods as an important way to signify one's social status in the expanding middle class. Breward (1995) describes the democratization of fashion through industry production as the cornerstone, through which clothing became the most accessible way for the middle class to display wealth and status: consumer culture emerged. On the other hand, larger scale display of weath could be achieved through homeownership and personal property. Especially in suburban areas, that were getting increasingly anonymous, architecture and housing became potent status symbols reflecting economic success (Jackson, 1985). Mobility, through automobiles, would distinguish individuals in the suburban environment, especially because now, owning a personal vehicle was a desired achievement (Flink, 1975); notably, vehicles had never been a tool for leisure before but used to be tools for agriculture. Personal leisure mobility on the other hand would now go along with another important status marker in middle class: *time*. As a sign of higher status, spending time off work would display a particular position in social hierarchy, because not needing to work all the time was something only some could afford. Thus, vacations and hobbies, according to Rojek (1995), were novel signs of status as well.

One of the most potent drivers for consumer culture was marketing and especially the introduction of advertising. As they became more sophisticated, and especially tailored to individuals from middle class, they would foster the desire to own status symbols, because they were now being increasingly associated with higher standing. The advent of mass media with newspapers, radio and TV brought forth celebrities who gained validation in wide social circles, way beyond immediate realm, through the ever-widening reach. Melting celebrity status and advertising would become an even more potent driver for consumption through the association it would build. The creation of an aspirational social image and class amplified the needs in individuals to not only distinguish themselves from the rest, but would link personal identity immediately to consumption patterns and create a perception of success and taste through owning certain products. Advertising was gradually becoming a tool for more than only selling products, because it created *brand loyalty* through branding products, in combination with the image conveyed by owning them. The created cultural narrative of purchasing reinforced the public image of achievement and personal identity got increasingly associated with the consumption of certain goods and brands (Habermas, 1989; Leiss et al., 1986; Leiss et al., 2005; Baudrillard, 1998; Frank, 1997; Marshall, 1977; Klein, 2000).

As industrialization progressed further, the described momentum laid the groundwork for modern forms of status anxiety through the compulsive seeking of social validation, because competition for social approval intensified exponentially. Two main reasons contributed to the birth of social pressure for validation and the increasing difficulty therein. The first one is the general rise of capitalism and with it, widening social circles: more public lives and a larger "audience" increased the initial pressure to display one's wealth and success, because, as the title of the chapter already suggests, moving from closeness to a large community brought forth a sense of competition in individuals in their desire to create marks of distinction. Growing cities and urbanization multiplicated the wideness of groups that could be potential *judges* on one's social status. Secondly, the expansion of the middle class in general brought along a growing number of people who got access to the same status symbols. Colloquially spoken, in a consumer society, where every family owns a house and a car, they are no longer status symbols but the new standard. That is, new status symbols had to be created or found, potentially ones that others could not easily achieve or afford (Thompson, 1963; Ewen, 1976; Goffman, 1959; Sennett, 1977; Baudrillard, 1998; Beck, 1992; Veblen, 1899).

In conclusion, industrialization created a strong momentum in consumer society with a strong desire for status markers of different kinds. By its progress and a growing number of members in the middle class however, competition arose, that would be hard to keep up with, since not only the stage for one's own personality and marks of distinction grew to large anonymous urban areas, but also the number of individuals with access to the same goods made them somewhat obsolete as means to distinguish oneself from the rest.

3.2   The Formation of Modern Global Citizenship

In the post-industrialization era, societies grew vastly and became more complex than ever before. Urbanization happened at a rapid pace and larger cities meant larger and more anonymous societies with increased social complexity (Giddens, 1990). In *The Rise of the Network Society*, Castells (2010) describes individuals in globalization, who seek social validation on a now global interconnected scale, through communication innovations and transportation simplification. It aligns with the views of Bauman (2007) and Turkle (2011), who found, that the expasnsion of postindustrial consumererism remained tied to purchasing power, brand loyalty and visibility on a global scale, but also with an increased speed in validation systems, which had shifted from local and national to global, and most importantly, as Rheingold (2000) concluded, in real-time. According to him, internet and the digital era, that accelerated global networks even more, created "arenas" for social validation. This can be described as a constant real-time competition for attention, in which individuals do not only feel the social pressure to perform before an incredibly large audience, but are constantly being judged against global social standards, which is a significant difference from the earlier forms of validation seeking in local communities – and of course even more different from being tied to increasing the chances of mere survival.

In this chapter, the main focus lies on the most significant differences between the digital era's forms of self-expression from *all* previous forms in the history of human evolution: While in earlier phases, social validation was constrained by proximity, limited to tangible indicators of success and status, none of the earlier stages afforded the opportunity for the extensive fabrication of identity that digital platforms now provide. The global reach of social media has extended the handling of approval far beyond immediate circles on the one hand, and on the other hand, digital forms of selfrepresentation introduced a critical transformation in how we present and validate our identites. For the first time in history, it enabled individuals to craft a curated identity that may differ markedly from their offline persona. Digital performance stages with digital audiences allow individuals groundbreaking opportunities to selectively emphasize certain aspects of themselves while downplaying others. Unlike all the previous stages, social media eventually provided the opportunity to fabricate an identity, by managing its entire narrative to the desired portrayal. Consequently, the lives and personalities portrayed online are idealized through the strategically enhanced best social version, with the validation received being based on the aspects individuals carefully choose to show and highlight. Likewise, new metrics of validation, also entirely digital, have likely outweighed traditional indicators for some. At a later point, I will elaborate on how these dynamics reinforce the showcasing of increasingly refined personas, with often unrealistic representations, capable of overshadowing individuals' true selves, regardless of their authenticity.

The facilitation of identity curation, with an expansive reach of social affirmation through online platforms has been extensively examined. Turkle (2011) has explored the techniques and abilities of individuals to manage their online personas, while they often do not accurately reflect their offline selves. This phenomenon, often referred to as the "representation of self" in digital contexts, reflects the willfull sharing of selective information and imagery to construct an idealized version of oneself (Goffman, 1959; Hogan, 2010). While Boyd (2014) and Van Dijck (2013) found, that the globalization of information distribution and the growing scale of validation create an increasing pressure for ongoing approval, Marwick & Boyd (2011) describe the difficulties in navigating the curation of information shared, in alignment with the varying expectations from diverse audiences. Accordingly, the idealized representation of oneself is mainly driven by the internal desire for modern forms of approval – digital affirmation (Chou & Edge, 2012; Marwick, 2013). Those new metrics used in the digital era serve as benchmarks for social worth (Gillespie, 2014; Van Dijck, 2013): this significant shift has fundamentally altered the way that individuals assess their own social standing against others and importantly, the emphasis on digital metrics over traditional status indicators. Abidin (2016) and Twenge (2018) suggest, that the introduction of these metrics, together with the growing reliance on them, contributes to manifold psychological effects in individuals, often adverse ones.

3.3 Overloading the Social Feedback System: The Disconnect Between Ancient Adaptations and Modern Society

A central question in this work is the extent to which social evolution has advanced to a level that surpasses the capacity of our inherent evolutionary framework. The exponential growth of social networks presents new opportunities for connection and affrirmation, yet also exerts considerable pressure on the systems our ancestors established for social validation. With increasing size and complexity, and at growing speeds, individuals have to navigate through large numbers of relationships and expectations. I mentioned earlier, that it could be observed, that the principle of socializing eventually found its way into our genetics, because early humans quickly internalized the need for communal proximity, and I raised the question whether the extent of social evolution has also shifted our cognitive systems in a similar manner – to easily handle the array of feedback we receive and manage the globality of connections and social pressure we are constantly under nowadays. Spoiler alert: No, it has not.

As we investigate the shifts in social evolution, it becomes evident, that our ancient cognitive limitations, inherently designed for smaller social circles, are encountering significant, and unprecented, challenges. This leads us to one of the foundational theories that provide insight into the cognitive constraints humans experience in this context: *Dunbar's number.*

Introduced by reputable anthropologist Robin Dunbar (1992; 1993), Dunbar's number refers to the theoretical cognitive limit of stable social connections a human individual can maintain, mainly limited by the size of the human neocortex. The research on primates' brain sizes and their corresponding social groups suggested, that there was a theoretical capability limit in processing social information and maintaining relationships, as well as comprehending group dynamics. Dunbar found, that similarly, there was a theoretical limitation for such in humans, depending on the size of the human neocortex in the brain. According to his estimates, humans can manage approximately 150 stable social relationships. While several studies made thereafter supported observable clusters around the figure (Hill & Dunbar, 2003; Sutcliffe et al., 2012), it remains subject of ongoing research in how far the size of the neocortex imposes the limitations responsible for this observed cluster, and what other factors might determine it, e. g. cultural and environmental influences.

However, in the context of contemporary social validation patterns, Dunbar's research underscores the significant discrepancy between modern scales of digital social networks and our cognitive capacities and limitations. With early social feedback stemming from immediate proximity in intimate familiar and local social circles, feedback remained manageable from emotional and also cognitive perspectives, since it was direct and personal. As has been established before, the digital era has significantly transformed this, far exceeding the number proposed by Dunbar. It is especially the exponential nature of growth, that our brains could not by any means have had the time to adapt to. The result are large numbers of superficial relationships, that however put pressure on the brain's ability to nurture meaningful relationships and adapt to feedback.

As a result of this shift, it may be suggested, that while individuals strive to exhibit themselves to a very large audience, their cognitive and emotional resources are insufficient for coping with the challenges of maintaining these networks from the perspective of manegement of social validation. Dunbar's findings suggest, that although our social brains have evolved to flourish in small and close social environments, the exponentially rapid growth of our networks and the pressure to adapt have outstripped our capacities to sustain a healthy processing of social validation.

Much unlike earlier eras, today's social feedback mechanisms are immediate. The novel forms of feedback and validation significantly alter the experience of social interaction in comparison to all previous periods of human history. Social platforms like Twitter, Instagram and Facebook have emerged as the key venues for identity affirmation (Boyd & Ellison, 2007), because they provide instant feedback in a direct connection to the content that is shared by a user. This creates a pattern of cause and effect with immediacy (Pempek et al., 2009), further supporting the habit of sharing highly selective information that provides the most, or the best, feedback. The permanent accessibility contrasts sharply with more localized and slow forms of approval that characterized previous societies. According to Valkenburg & Peter (2011), the perpetual availability fosters certain behaviors in users, that become fully integrated in their daily lives. Based on these habits, social platforms have long established sophisticated mechanisms, that foster perpetual user engagement in order to prolong the time spent with the platforms, for monetary reasons (Bucher, 2012; Gross, 2023; Gross et al., 2024). Furthermore, in my (2024) work *Cognitive Nemesis*, I have described how algorithmic curation of content and the human psychological susceptibility work in perfect unison to create an ever-perpetuated loop. However, this work is not primarily focused on the mechanisms behind social media, even though they contribute much to the behavioral patterns that many individuals exhibit nowadays.

Ellison et al. (2006) found, that social platforms enable users to craft and display carefully constructed identities for the audience, with each update sophisticatedly curated to reflect the certain aspects of the persona that they want to exhibit. According to research by Lomborg (2013) and Gerlitz & Helmond (2013), the simultaneous use of multiple such platforms enhances these dynamics further, allowing individuals to seek validation across various digital spaces, each defined by their own metrics, but creating a comparable manner – and an overwhelming experience, most certainly adding to the cognitive load. Moreover, as mentioned before, the perpetual nature of the platforms, along with their accessibility and the ever-widening social circles they amplify, there is a certain atmosphere of competition through the visibility of others' validation metrics. This blends perfectly into Adler's theories, which will be explained later on. Vogel et al. (2014) identified, that social comparison is significantly heightened by the visibility of peers' metrics, while according to studies from the Pew Research Center (2018), the permanent pursuit of social approval is specifically reinforced through real-time notifications, that keep users in a state of reactive alertness. This, according to Robinson (2017), leads to behavioral patterns of validation seeking, that are gradually exhibited *outside* of specific contexts, which is a particularly important finding. The behaviors of continuous validation-seeking, amplified by modern digital environments, become an ongoing presence in users' lives. It particularly the absence of downtime in digital spaces which nowadays contributes to the mental strain in users; while historically, social interactions would leave an individual the time to rest, used for processing and reflection, the current digital environments lack any pause and cause a permanent oversaturation of social input (Alter, 2017; Carr, 2010; Rainie & Wellman, 2012). According to Crawford (2015), one of the consequences of this is the lack of prioritization of feedback, due to the cognitive overload it creates. Marwick (2013) and Gillespie (2018) conclude, that the real-time tracking of validation metrics exacerbates the pressure for public performance through continually managing the online presence to what is believed to be ideal.

In this chapter, I want to mention another concern particularly present in digital landscapes. Social validation is increasingly reduced to measurable metrics of engagement, such as likes and follower numbers. This trend does not only mean a quantitative, but also qualitative shift of receiving social approval, without any historical precedent. As has been clarified, historically, the social feedback mechanisms were built on direct interaction and provided social signals that an individual could interpret. With a transition to numerical assessments, where an individual can gauge their social standing in real-time and through numerical data, there is no evolutionary basis for any cognitive processing of such. Through the dry and computational quantification of social approval, the brain lacks the evolutionary makeup to process quantitative social data, let alone continuous streams of it. Consequently, individuals experience cognitive challenges as they have to manage not only the quality of their relationships, but also the fluctuating metrics now defining their social standing at any given time. However, there is no emotional context that the human mind is equipped with in assigning meaningful and experience-based interpretations of rather abstract metrics like modern ones. Persistent exposure to quantified social data can mean tremendous pressure for individuals, since the "social validation terminal" is always up to date and publicly visible; divorced to a large extent from any authentic human interaction that is genetically accessible. It can be argued, that our cognitive capacities have never been designed for anything near those amounts and steady flows of social pressure.

According to Marwick & Boyd (2011), individuals nowadays manage multiple personas simultaneously, with each one tailored to a distinct audience, which causes a huge cognitive load through fragmentation of personality aspects, that have to be adapted and disrupts individuals' selfperception. In alignment with those findings, Kross et al. (2013) argue, that conflicting expectations and feedback streams exacerbate the fragmentation of identities that people manage, predominantly because people expect praise and criticism based on displayed aspects of their personas and the specific audience. Meeting divergent expectations across various platforms is a mental task, that demands constant management; the human brain has no precedent in such activities throughout history, hence the permanent alertness and pressure causes significant cognitive loads (Walther et al., 2008). Accordingly, Roberts & David (2020) found, that those behaviors potentially cause mental stress and specific anxiety, confirming the findings from Berryman et al. (2018), who argue, that self-doubt, anxiety and mental stress are the result of the perpetual mental burden of managing distinct personas and identities in the digital world. I want to add, that oftentimes, balancing audience-targeted personas is a walk on thin ice, since the delicate balances that are needed to maintain consistent and coherent images of oneself across various displays can lead to incompatible aspects in identity. Ultimately, the cognitive dissonance it can create in individuals, specifically when the portrayed persona does not match the intrinsic beliefs and convictions has been one of the key topics in my former publication *Cognitive Nemesis*. This aligns with findings by Heatherton (2011), who describes the brain's inherent desire for coherence, which, in this context, is especially disrupted in self-perception, because reconciling conflicting and inconsistent social feedback is particularly difficult to process for us, and these issues are multiplied across all the publicly visible feedback streams.

4 THE MECHANISMS OF MODERN SOCIAL FEEDBACK OVERLOAD

4.1 Media and Advertising: The Construction of Idealized Social Standards

As established earlier, the emergence of the middle class during the era of industrialization led to the development of status symbols with individuals increasingly expressing their social standing through the display of wealth and material possessions. Especially fashion, housing and personal assets were important external markers of success. This era represented an important transformation in how social standing was perceived.

As advertising evolved alongside the rise of consumer culture, it played an important role in reinforcing these status symbols, establishing a direct connection between materialism and social approval. The cultural narrative of consumption as a means of achieving social validation from peers continued to grow exponentially, with mass media enhancing the external visibility of these markers significantly. Especially the strategy of employing particularly aspirational figures like celebrities were utilized to create emotional connections and promote idealized lifestyles associated with certain brands and products.

In the contemporary digital era, these dynamics are stronger than ever before, and are increasingly intensifying. While traditional status symbols still possess a high social value in contemporary culture, there have been new, additional indicators of success, that are original to the digital era. Here is the melting pot, where modern phenomena and the established mechanisms of external validation intertwine: advertising and social media foster social landscapes, that idealize showcased lifestyles to an often absurd degree – be it beauty standards, wealth, social circles or whatever else but also, the aforementioned idealized personas that users create of themselves. The unattainable ideal is perpetuated on both sides; users are presented and internalize perfection in every manner, perpetually, and also, they present the most idealized form of themselves and broadcast it into the digital world.

These phenomena are the ones that will be explained in detail in this chapter; with a particular focus on how the permanent ongoing and still growing idealization of life brings forth new social standards and dynamics that people nowadays live by, how they trick us into permanent upwards comparisons and how they create even more needs of social validation. After that, these dynamics will be observed through the lens of the *Inferiority Complex* introduced by Alfred Adler, and how they influence our self-perception.

Williams (1980) and Kilbourne (1999) describe, how advertising and television gradually became pivotal in reflecting cultural norms and societal expectations and thereby shaping public perception of ideals, creating idealized lifestyles and personas, that the audience would internalize. The visual element of television created compelling and powerful forms of advertising, that transported narratives of aspirational lives and social roles, and connected them with certain products. According to Leiss et al. (1986), it was particularly the power of visual representation that made the message so effective. It was also then, that a broader public would not only gain access to material wealth, but that the image of wealth, success and social standing was continually reinforced in order to sell products and brands. The strategy worked well, especially since during the rise of the middle class, people would take part in the ongoing competition for attention and reflection of their social standing through purchasing power. According to Ewen (1976) and Marchand (1985), the portrayal of the "good life extended well beyond the advertising of the mere product, because it conveyed the way of life, that people *should* aspire for: through shaping societal expectations, the transported message was clear. The ideal way of life was what was shown on television, and advertising gave people the instruction how to achieve it. The constructed image centered around material wealth and its display as a visual representation of social status – triggering the inherent sense of approval and belonging in audiences. Schudson (1984) found, that this method encouraged viewers to align their personal virtues with the portrayed ones, especially in terms of consumption. Similarly, Goldman & Papson (1996) describe, how the established connection between material wealth and consumption with the idealized form of society and individual way of life worked in the way, that individuals quickly adopted the narrative of linking material success to social approval.

These findings present a clear image of the progression of society, divorcing their self-perception and social aspirations from intrinsic and rather private values towards the public image they wanted to maintain, which was mainly through the exhibition of material possessions. Advertising can be described as a particularly strong force, because it would set the standards for aspirational lifestyles and contributed significantly to what consumers perceived as the social standards they would strive to achieve. Through this, advertising was much more than only the promotion of products, it became a source of inspiration and even the social instance for the design of an idealized society, and through that determined the place each individual aspired for themselves in this construction. In their 1995 work *Liberatory postmodernism and the reenchantment of consumption*, Firat & Venkatesh explain, how television with its advertisings created standardized images and perceptions of success, and consequently, individuals increasingly measured their own self-worth against the showcased ideals, relying more and more on the external validation from the public. The notable shift is described in their chapter *Modernist Construction of the Consumption/Production Dichotomy and the Beginnings of the Postmodern Critique:*

> [...] Consumption was regarded as secondary to production. It did not create anything of significant (i.e., economic) value for society or humanity. [...] Consumption was only to replentish the individual to carry out the really important, meaningful – thus valuable activities in the public domain. [...] (p. 245).

Later on, they draw on Douglas & Isherwood (1979), and find, that

> Douglas and Isherwood go on to show how in various domains of consumption, such as food, clothing and various other goods, activities become highly symbolic acts that are invested with meanings derived from cultural frameworks. Goods become means of conveying messages among individuals and groups of individuals. (pp. 248-249).

In a younger work, Holt (2002) describes television advertising as a meaningful contributor to the understanding of social norms and their evolution, especially regarding success, identity and materialism, which still influences modern-day perceptions of social validation. The effect however is not only individuals' alignment of virtues and aspirations with the portrayed lifestyles. Prevailing standards in subsets like beauty, wealth and success create an environment of competition, as has been explained, with necessarily fostering dichotomies. Those who fall behind those standards, feel inadequate. Frith et al. (2005) were able to find, that beauty standards in advertising have been pafrticularly narrow, favoring Eurocentric ideals and marginalizing diverse body types, and exacerbating feelings of inadequacy among those individuals who did not conform with these standards. Similarly, in a much earlier work, Jhally (1987) describes, how reinforcement of social norms through repetitive showcasing of *flawless, perfect, happy and successful* individuals contribute to consumer dissatisfaction with their own lives.

These triggers of dissatisfaction have not only been planted in consumers, but they were intended: if an ideal is established as a common standard, and is widely accepted, the social validation need in individuals would be a mighty component in making a purchasing decision. The conveyed message was clear: *'You do not meet the standard (yet), you need to buy the product'*. Triggering a sense of insecurity in consumers and converting it into a purchasing decision through the establishment of an unattainable standard can be described as a sophisticated marketing trick, while I don't make any moral judgement at this point. Especially women have historically been the target of such planted insecurities by presentations of 'perfect' skin, hair, bodies and overall beauty standards. Linked with a perceived sense of happiness, consumption was subtly undetachably melted with a happier life and personal fulfillment. Likewise, the reinforcement of certain social hierarchies can be perceived as a casualty, by marginalizing individuals who did not fit these ideals (Tiggemann & McGill, 2004; Richins, 1991; Berger, 1972).

Media advertising has always needed these standards. With rising mass production in the industrialization era, and a growing consumer base (middle class), the drive for social validation and admiration was the strongest factor in fostering purchasing decisions. The strategic depiction of flawless individuals became a powerful tool to invoke an aspiration based on an inherent trait of the human psyche. Using celebrities would become the bridge for that aspiration: the message conveyed was that the product granted access to a more socially desirable lifestyle. In his groundbreaking 1954 work, Festinger describes, how the individual comparison with the portrayed perfection is the exact desired mechanism at play. Based on his observations, advertising relies on the strategy to make consumers compare themselves to idealized standards, necessarily creating a gap. This gap would then consequently be bridged through possession of the product advertised. Festinger (1954) argues:

> When a discrepancy exists with respect to opinions or abilities there will be tendencies to change one's own position so as to move closer to others in the group (Derivation D_l, p. 126).

and

> The stronger the attraction to the group the stronger will be the pressure toward uniformity concerning abilities and opinions within that group (Corollary VII A, p. 131).

From these important deductions, it can be concluded, that the particular attraction mentioned before is indeed planted and carefully constructed, since not only the attraction of a seemingly *perfect* life is strong, it becomes much stronger through its establishment as a societal *standard* – there is a particular element of the fear of exclusion (think of ancestry here), if an individual fails to meet the standard. The conveyed easily attainable bridge (the product) becomes the new means of aspiration, through equalizing it with the element of inclusion.

In preparation for the next chapter, where we will take a closer look onto the perpetual cycles of upward comparisons, we will briefly investigate the latest stage of portrayed idealization in the digital era, and the changes it has brought to the dynamics, especially in advertising. A significant observartion I would like to share is that one of the primary distinctions between traditional advertising and contemporary media lies in the transition from passive to active engagement.

While historically, audiences were presented with advertisements on predefined schedules (in television), this means a passive manner of consumption of the promoted idealized lifestyles. In contrast, today's digital environments encourage users to actively seek out and engage with content from influencers. Through subscriptions, following and the active consumption of content, viewers are no more just passively presented with the idealized social standards they would internalize; they willingly and actively engage with the content. Influencers have merged the curated perfection with entertainment, meaning that the promoted ideals have become an integral aspect of the overall entertainment experience. The active immersion with these narratives is a significant shift in the presentation of unattainable perfection; the active pursuit of content and the encouragement thereof is an element that passive reception of conventional advertising lacked.

Building on this thought, I want to expand on the perceived proximity of influencers to their audiences. While influencers held a minor role in the marketing sphere in the beginning, they have now emerged as formidable advocates for brands and products. From what we can perceive today, this appears to be a significant paradigm shift, because of several reasons. Historically, advertising presented by aspirational figures like actors or musicians or other mega-celebrities, they were distant and unattainable. Together with the previously discussed passive element of advertising, the shift becomes clear: on the one hand, there has been a significant transformation from passive reception to active engagement with the content, through the merging of the actual content consumed and the lifestyle promoted. The advertising becomes an active ingredient in the entertainment, which is actively chosen, clicked, consumed by the audience. Moreover, it is particularly the very fact, that influencers do *not* have the lofty status of mega-celebrities, decreasing the perceived distance and maintaining accessibility. Although they can acquire a substantial social reach nowadays – *which, as we remember, has become an aspirational status symbol of its own!* – they bridge the gap between unreachable celebrities and everyday individuals much more effectively, conveying the 'one of us'-

narrative. The promoted lifestyles become more relatable and through direct interaction and connections, the environment becomes vividly immersive, tangible and perceivedly achievable. These environments, whether in fashion, beauty or technology, engage audiences in new ways that traditional passive advertising never could.

While all these thoughts can be well-explained, there are many reasons, why the shift has only been in the transportation and consumption of the content, but not in the degree of idealizing social lifestyles and status. On the contrary; contemporary research shows, that the extent of fabrication has increased significantly through digital media and has reached new highs. Chou & Edge (2012) argue, that the frequent and widespread use of photo editing tools, filters and selective sharing create an idealized representation of overall reality, which significantly distorts users' perceptions of what is attainable or typical. It is a common observation, that specifically those accounts that achieve a substantial social reach make extensive use of edited material, which is then adopted among individual private users. It is arguable, which feelings of anxiety it would create among heavy users of social media platforms to share each authentic aspect of their lives, including those that they might supposedly lessen their social validation, and what feelings it would invoke if they shared unedited photos of themselves to their audiences. However, influencers play a key role in promoting and maintaining these hyperreal standards through the sophisticated curation of their contents and the careful editing of the idealized and controlled versions of their lives, often for profit (Abidin, 2016). This curation reaches the desired goal; according to Dumas et al. (2017), it leads to blurred lines between authenticity and performance, creating the impression that influencers live flawless lives, filled only with desirable activities and achievements, standards and reinforcing unrealistic impressions and measures of sucess, paired with the absence of any negative connotations or failure. Tiggemann & Slater (2013) found, that the extensive use of photo editing and filters perpetuate unrealistic and unattainable beauty standards that solely rely on digital manipulation.

In episode no. 33 of their podcast *ikario*, Oliver Cowlishaw and Shane Melaugh talk about the 'Instagram Face', which is a novel term, prominent all over the internet, relating to a perceived trend revolving around the app 'Face Tune': they describe, how according to famous celebrity makeupartist Colby Smith, the vast majority of the most followed people on Instagram use the app. In their explanation, Face Tune is an artificial intelligence which detects a face in an uploaded picture and is capable of altering facial features without deeper knowledge of photo editing or skills with sophisticated photo editing software. They further cite Smith saying that of those, which he claims to be 95% (*Smith's own approximation; may be dramatized*), most individuals had had some kind of cosmetic surgery, of which most followed specific trends (e. g. lifted eyebrows). The really interesting part of their argumentation is, that the dynamics of beauty standards have shifted from merely seeing what is perceived as a beautiful face, and subsequently aspiring to look similar, have shifted. Now, there is an algorithmic deterministic characterization of beauty, that is being reinforced through the modern metrics attached to it, with the clear message of 'This is the look of success, and you should replicate it' – because obviously – measurably – there is numerical success derived from that certain look. Shane Melaugh elaborates:

> It's an A.I. that detects your face and you can then just use some simple slide or say like give me fuller lips, give me longer lashes, give me narrower cheekbones or whatever it is, right. So you just have a bunch of slides and it does it automatically. It's basically like a Photoshop program where you don't have to actually learn Photoshop, because it just detects the features of your face and you can manipulate them [...]. And he basically says, look, of all the celebrities on Instagram and the people with the most followers, he [Smith] says,

easily 95% use Face Tune. So you're not seeing their real face, you're seeing their face after it's been tuned. He also says 'and I would say that 95% people all have also had some sort of cosmetic procedure; you can see things trending, like everyone's getting brow-lifts by Botox now'. And again, here's how this ties in with everything we've talked about before: the normal story that we're usually told about this is that yes, there are some beauty standards, you know, and of course some people will aspire to look similar, but what's the harm. But there are a couple of factors here that I think are easily overlooked. One is, that there is this algorithmic incentive and reinforcement: it's not just people looking at pictures and going 'Oh, this is a really nice looking face, I wish my face looked like this' – no. It is an algorithm surfacing and incentivizing a certain look. So there's a certain look, that will get more likes, more comments, more reach, more sponsorships, etc. It is more attention, more reach and more money in a certain look over another look. And so that adds a completely different factor into this equation. It is not just 'I'm looking at someone that looks prettier than me'. It is 'This person, or this kind of face' – and that's where we see the convergence – 'is the famous Instagram influencer lifestyle riches face. This kind of face is the everything I want in life face.' And also with that conversion where the algorithm is creating that convergence – because, of two things, again – you have a signal being boosted; other people who are incentivized, they're basically coping this, they also want to be Instagram famous, they also want validation, they also want to be an Instagram influencer, are seeing a repetition of this kind of style, this kind of picture, and so they want to do more of that. And the more of that, the more of the similar thing is in the system, the more likely it is – this is the algorithmic bias – that the algorithm goes 'Oh, this kind of thing is popular, so I should show it to more people.' and it becomes self-reinforcing. And Face Tune is an imperfect program. Face Tune is a program that looks at a picture and identified the things that are the easiest to identify about a face; and it will be differently able to make changes to different features of a face. And it will be most able to just exaggerate some obvious features like big lashes, big lips and so on. And so, even Face Tune itself contributes to what the Instagram Face ends up looking like. Like, if there is a parallel dimension, where Face Tune is a bit different, like a bit differently capable, the U.I. is a bit different – and we end up with a different Instagram Face. Because of that. That's my point. And people are getting plastic surgery to look like this. Okay? This is how it's reaching out into the real world; people are getting plastic surgery and what's literally happening – I read this in an article as well, where a plastic surgeon was like 'what's normal, what used to be is that clients come in with a picture of an actress or something and say 'I want a nose like her'; now, people come in with a picture of themselves that they face-tuned and say 'I want to look like this.' (Podcast *ikario*, Episode 33, Minute 30:37-35:34).

In 2018, Kleemans et al. argued, that the level of fabrication in social media has escalated, heightening social expectations and promoting new comparison habits, hat weren't known in other eras. Similarly, Fardouly et al. (2015) found, that the seemingly perfect existences of influencers lead consumers to dissatisfaction with their own lives. Moreover, the swap into real life has been found to be significant, as the constant curation and establishment of hyperreal representations of life appears to impact traditional notions of authenticity and self-representation (Ellison et al., 2007).

In conclusion, advertising is a potent medium for reinforcing status symbols, connecting consumerism with individuals' emotionally charged social desires. The trend of idealization has significantly intensified in the digital era, especially through the introduction of new social markers such as likes, followers and curated personas emerging on social platforms. However, although the pursuit of social validation is a long-standing human trait, social media has introduced novel challenges with its metrics and understanding of social approval. The unparalleled influx of social feedback compels users to engage in constant self-assessment and validation-seeking behavior, often to absurd levels. Consequently, social approval itself has become a desirable status symbol, because the digital real-time indicators are publicly visible.

The tricky part of modern social validation lies in its distribution through public personas, that, unlike distant and unattainable mega-celebrites are often viewed as much closer and authentic. It is especially this relatability, the 'just like the average person'-type of online persona, that reinforces the authenticity of idealized lifestyles and social standards so effectively. While the perceived lifestyles appear more tangible through the proximity asnd intimacy these influencers convey, it does not change the fact, that their curated lives are not authentic and do not represent an attainable standard. With these foundations established, we will now examine the rise of constant upward comparison, as a means to shed more light on the psychological and potential neurochemical impacts.

4.2 Social Media and the Escalation of Upward Comparison

The phenomenon of upward comparison is not original to the digital era. It has been observed for decades and has also been subject of manifold studies in human psychology and sociology. However, the fact that in modern times, we observe downright absurd forms of comparison among individuals makes it a timely actual topic, especially in approaches to explain modern social dynamics and their psychological impacts on individuals and groups.

In his groundbreaking 1954 work *A Theory of Social Comparison Processes*, Festinger introduced his ideas on the human characteristic to possess an intrinsic motivation to assess their own abilities, opinions and their overall worth. Festinger argues, that these traits are crucial for the development of own identity. He observed, that humans have the inherent drive to diminish states of uncertainty concerning their own abilities and behaviors by comparing themselves to similar peers. This form of comparison yields a 'relative assessment' of success or failure, which aids individuals in their evaluation of their self-worth across numerous contexts. A key aspect of Festinger's theory is that the inherent drive in individuals does not favor social comparison over other means of assessment, but in absence of any objective, non-social benchmark, humans tend to compare themselves to others with similar features. In other words, in social scenarios, where there are no definitive and comprehensive standards, for example beauty, success or social relationships, individuals still need to assess their own worth and thus naturally rely on comparison with others. According to Festinger, this assessment provides direction and important social information, as well as a sense of affirmation (think success vs. failure). The publication of this theory garnered considerable acknowledgement and confirmation among scientists and still provides important foundational insights in human behavior and its frameworks for social dynamics. For instance, studies by Wills (1981) and Buunk & Ybema (1997), that are concerned with upward and downward comparisons as means of self-evaluation found, that these significantly impact self-concept, social interactions and emotional well-being.

In this chapter, we will specifically examine the phenomenon of upward comparison and how it is an important driving fac-

tor in modern social dynamics, specifically when perceived
through the lens of digital networks, and we will assess the
psychological foundations in the greater context of social feedback overload and the overstimulation and oversaturation with
expectations and self-assessment.

In the context of self-improvement, the comparison with
other individuals leads to a pushing mechanism to achieve
more and perform better, refining one's self-perception. Wood
(1989) argues, that comparisons with others can foster personal growth through motivation for improving. This aligns
with the knowledge about the early stages of cognitive development, where comparison takes a pivotal role. Bandura's
(1977) *Social Learning Theory*, a widely acknowledged framework for the understanding of cognitive learning mechanisms
in children, posits, that observation and adaptation are critical elements of learning skills and behaviors, validating the
general narrative, that individuals use self-assessment in comparison with peers to learn through imitation and adaptation. Although a significant portion of learning is achieved
through direct instruction by more capable peers, children use
their observation and direct comparison of their own abilities
to learn. Similarly, the so-called *Zone of Proximal Development*, a framework developed by Vygotsky (1978), explains,
that children in their developmental stages use comparison
to more capable peers to identify areas of own improvement
and the abilities they want to learn through guidance. The
proximity is an important element, because it helps children
gauge their own assessments through direct interaction with
others, comparing their own status quo to those around them.
The findings have been confirmed in numerous studies (Harter, 1983; Schunk, 1987) and can be directly linked to established knowledge on identity formation processes. As Markus
& Wurf (1987) posit, the self-concept, which is an ongoing
and continuously evolving dynamic understanding of the self,
is significantly shaped by comparisons with peers. Thereby,
social evolution can be seen as never finished in an individual;
the identity shaping social life is refined through interactions

lifelong. Building on that, we understand social comparison does not occur in isolation. It is deeply tied to group dynamics, and we know, that human beings derive a significant portion of their sense of self and their identity formation from the groups they belong to. According to Tajfel & Turner (1979) and their *Social Identity Theory*, individuals develop an in-group and an out-group identity, which also shapes collective understanding of the group; the collective identity. This is particularly interesting in light of further studies conducted by Crocker & Luthanen (1990), who found, that the collective identification with the in-group is particularly beneficial for individuals' self-esteem if they belong to a high-status group. This adds layers of complexity to the own identity, because the aspect of belonging to a desirable collective enhances the self-assessment. Accordingly, group membership can lead to positive assessments of the self and consequently 'ease' social comparison.

Humans appear to have inherited these self-assessment mechanisms from tribal age, deeply embedding them into their genetic code. In early human societies, peer influence and adaptation was not only socially desirable, but an important means for survival, therefore, humans would quickly inherit these traits of social learning as survival strategies (Henrich & Gil-White, 2001; Tomasello, 2014; Boehm, 1999; Humphrey, 1976). Furthermore, as Deci & Ryan (1985) describe, the survival-based comparison, embedded in human nature, fosters a lifelong drive for self-improvement and adaptation to challenges, which helps individuals meet societal and personal expectations; nowadays just as it did in tribal age.

When individuals compare themselves to others they perceive as superior, this can essentially trigger two different psychological mechanisms. On the one hand, the perceived superiority of others, particularly their abilities or achievements oneself is lacking, can function as an important driver for own motivation. On the other hand, it can also invoke feelings of inadequacy (Festinger, 1954). Through comparing themselves with others, that appear to have achieved more or are performing better, humans have a tendency to raise their own standards, which can be a powerful drive for the motivation to strive toward reaching those standards themselves. However, albeit triggering self-reflection, the identification of prevailing gaps between what they define as ideal and their own current persona, can lead not only to motivation, but also frustration, depending on the target and the gap itself (Collins, 1996; Mussweiler et al., 2004). I would like to highlight, that in this context, we should recall the gap that is perceived between the lives humans live and the curated lives that are represented in digital ages. It is logical, that the perceived gaps are enormous, if an individual is constantly presented with the 'perfect' lives of other 'average' persons; yet, the own life can not measure up to those by any means. Herein lies the danger for the own cognitive processing: if all that we see is others, who have no hardships in life, who earn absurd sums of money, can virtually afford anything, while they are absurdly pretty, muscular or whatever, have perfect friends and nothing ever goes wrong; how are we expected to live up to those standards, because all we know from our previous life experience is, that however hard we try, we are never getting anywhere near such 'perfect' lives. Thus, this *gap* that we identify is *impossible to bridge*, for all we know. How should this not lead to frustration, but motivation, if all we have ever learned about our own lives contradicts the logic of ever attaining such perfection? The only logical conclusion we can derive from seeing these impressions, over and over, must be: there are uncountably many persons that are better at everything, and we should not even try, because we have zero chance.

I would like to expand deeper on this thought. When modern upward social comparison is coupled with the perpetual exposure to carefully curated representation of seemingly perfect lives, lived by personas who appear to excel in virtually everything, there can be an outcome of a much wider gap, a diminished equilibrium between motivation and frustration. As it is widely undertood, that we do only see the positive highlights of others' lives, what we need to address is the gap between our perception of what we believe is ideal – which is, of course, a product of curation, and is perpetually reinforced – and our own lived experiences. Because despite our best efforts, we find ourselves unable to attain these perfect outcomes – from the experience we have been living for all of our lives. If, like we have established before, the main two triggered mechanisms of upward comparison are motivation and frustration, in other words the aspiration to perform equally, and the frustration stemming from the realization that we don't, or won't, there is no more equilibrium between those. From all we have experienced, failure is a part of trying; but obviously not for others. They live what we have internalized as the desirable ideal. And for them, it goes smoothly. As far as we see. Despite unrealistic, we are constantly reinforced with the narrative of '*they* can do it' – but from our experience, we can not. For us, failure has always been part of life. When these two incompatible cognitive realizations collide, there is only one possible outcome. Our experience contradicts the possibility, that we can ever achieve such flawless perfection; however, other individuals proudly display exactly that. Thus, we must end up with the conclusion, that *the others* are just *better*, and this is indeed a frustrating conclusion to make.

When Leon Festinger (1957) introduced his concept of Cognitive Dissonance, he found, that if there are conflicting or contradicting thoughts, beliefs, convictions or behaviors in individuals, they experience discomfort. The discomfort triggers them to seek to reestablish an inner equilibrium, by either changing own behaviors or convictions, or by altering beliefs, so that there is a coherence in logic. This framework of rationality and emotions is a highly regarded explanation for human behavior in conflicting situations, or when beliefs and reality seem to collide.

It can be perfectly applied to the prevailing psychological mechanism described before: if what we see is perfection in others, which is constantly reinforced to us, we would of course like to achieve the same. However, based on our life experience, perfection is not realistic, because failure is inevitable part of trying. Those two realizations do not match, they are inconsistens; and we need to have an explanation as to why others seem to live a perfect life, but we can not, however hard we try, because the incoherent 'reality' that we are presented and our own reality seem to be two different, incompatible worlds. Therefore, the only logical conclusion we can derive will be: *I am just not good enough, and I will never be.* These ideas are supported by contemporary research on social media dynamics, such as Vogel et al. (2014), who found, that the repetitive exposure to the lived standards of others creates an initial motivation, quickly followed by the realization that it is a frustrating pursuit; leading to a gradual erosion of self-efficacy. Tiggemann & Slater (2013) similarly found, that the conclusion we draw from being reinforced that others excel while we fail, is that they are just 'better' and we will not ever be able to live up to such standards. Fardouly et al. (2015) see one of the key factors of the mental strain in the perpetuated confrontation with one's own limitations.

On the other hand, it has been found, that the opposite, downward comparison, can serve as a mechanism of protection against these dynamics. As a provider of psychological comfort, a comparison with individuals that are inferior to oneself in certain contexts, can enhance self-esteem through an affirmation of personal superiority. the protective mechanism lies in the shielding of the self-concept by focusing on others' failures or disadvantages (Wills, 1981; Aspinwall & Taylor, 1993). At a later point in this work, I want to share a brief elaboration on the question whether the comfort of superiority provided by downward social comparison can invoke *narcissistic* tendencies, just as the opposite – upward comparisons through perpetuated presentation of idealized social standards, as described above – can arguably lead to a reinforcement spiral of inferiority and dissatisfaction.

Before, I would like to briefly skim through the brain activity linked to the mechanisms in question, as to introduce the second main focal point of this work; an approach to the cognitive foundations of and possible derivations from modern social dynamics.

For the activity of the brain involved in social comparison, there are four areas we will analyze:
The Medial Prefrontal Cortex (mPFC), the Orbitofrontal Cortex (OFC), the *Dorsal Anterior Cingulate Cortex (dACC)* and the *Ventral Anterior Cingulate Cortex (vACC)*. On the following diagram, the location of each in the Neocortex and the transitional area between *Neocortex* and *Limbic Lobe* can be easily identified (note, that while 'rACC' and 'vACC' describe the same region here, rACC (rostral ACC) usually emphasizes the anterior positioning, while vACC (ventral ACC) emphasizes the lower part – for the visualization however, we can use them interchangeably in this case):

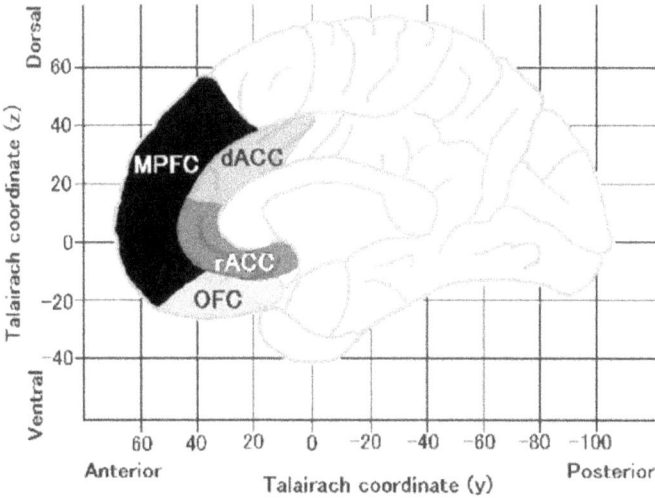

Figure 1: Schematic illustration of the locations of *mPFC*, *dACC*, *rACC* and *OFC* in the Prefrontal Cortex and around the Corpus Callosum (Nakao et al., 2009).

The roles and functions of the *mPFC* are quite impressive. It is essential for a range of sociocognitive processes and significantly influences individuals' perceptions, evaluations and responses to social stimuli. It is actively engaged in social comparison, showing activation during upward *and* downward comparison. Through this, it helps in modulation of social reactions to status (Luo et al., 2018). Additionally, the mPFC plays a significant role in evaluation of social hierarchies, because it affects assessments of the self and also other individuals, based on positional social standings. Furthermore, its influence in making social decisions has been highlighted (Koski et al., 2020). According to Molenberghs & Morrison (2014), it is further a key element in the recognition of group memberships, demonstrating increased activation in in-group member categorization processes. This is an important cue for its key function in social categorization and group dynamics. As we established earlier, humans learn and add layers to their identity formation through numerous social actions; the mPFC is a key element in the contribution to the regulation of own behavior based on the feedback received from peers (Seid-Fatemi & Tobler, 2015). The tendency to favor ingroup peers is another phenomenon, that points back at the influence of the mPFC; according to Volz et al. (2009), the mediation of empathy and heightened emotional potential in self-reference is particularly pronounced in the mPFC region of the brain. These findings strongly align with Euston et al.'s (2012) studies on the role of the mPFC in learning, particularly adaptative responses; they highlight how the mPFC plays a key role in associations between different contexts. In a 2023 study, Qu et al. used transcranial direct current stimulation (tDCS) and were able to prove the mPFC's involvement in learning about social ranks by observation. These findings suggest, that social hierarchies are learned through observation of peers under direct involvement of the mPFC. There is also evidence for a connectivity and direct interaction between the mPFC with the Amygdala region, in activation during social comparison processes, which suggests the interplay of emotional regulation processes in a parallel to upward or downward comparison in social dynamics (Jung & Kim, 2020). In a nuanced 2023 study, Kim et al. found, that the mPFC's subregions play distinctive roles in social adaptation scenarios; through fMRI data, it could be revealed, that the ventral, rostral and dorsal mPFC showed increased activity in the investigations of conformity to social hierarchies, in dependency of the individual's own perception of superiority or inferiority in the partners, general conforming tendencies and public or private contexts. The findings suggested the strategic role of the mPFC subregions in weighing scenarios against each other (e.g. exhibition of an increased probability of alignment with the preferences of a superior partner in a public setting), highlighting the important decision-making aspect of the mPFC in social environments and comparison settings. Lastly, I would like to highlight the studies conducted by J. Beer et al., that contribute significantly to the understanding of the mPFC and other brain regions in the particular context of social comparison and validation.

The mPFC is relevant for self-referential processing and evaluations related to the sense of self, in both abstract and in real-time contexts: it could be shown, that activation of the mPFC during processes of self-reflection highlights its prominent role in monitoring internal cues during self-evaluation and as well in those of others (i. e. judgment of personality traits) – either in relation to general qualities or in specific behaviors in social comparison (Beer & Hughes, 2009). In the same work, they were able to show how the mPFC is more active when people think about concrete contextual traits, which suggests that it helps processing self-representation, associating the mPFC with evaluations of the self in comparison to others. However, in diminishing biases (the so-called 'above-average effect'), the mPFC appears to play a minor role. Instead, it is suggested, that the *Orbitofrontal Cortex* (OFC) and the *dorsal Anterior Cingulate Cortex* (dACC) play more important roles in mediating biases in self-assessments; hence, these two have been mentioned before in particular. In other words, while the mPFC is a prominent actor in self-evaluation, it is the interplay with the OFC and the dACC, that calibrates overconfidence and reduces biased judgements. The aforementioned 'above-average effect' describes the tendency of individuals to assess their own capabilities at least better than average. I have drawn specific attention to this in my assessments of the Dunning-Kruger Effect in *Cognitive Nemesis*, explaining, that among other reaons, there has been systemic criticism against the long-established phenomenon Dunning and Kruger found; one of which is the postulated general tendency of individuals to perceive themselves as better than average – mathematically however, this is of course impossible (Kruger & Dunning, 1999; Magnus & Peresetsky, 2022; Gaze, 2023; Nuhfer, 2017 *in*: Gross, 2024). Interestingly, in their study *Roles of Medial Prefrontal Cortex and Orbitofrontal Cortex in Self-evaluation* (2010), Beer et al. found, that OFC and dACC showed decreased activation when individuals assessed themselves more positively, pointing at their involvement in mitigating overconfident self-assessments. Furthermore, it could be seen that OFC activity was diminished when easily available or irrelevant information bossted one's perceived performance, further solidifying the assumption that the OFC has significant involvement in avoiding biases that stem from one's own overconfidence. That is, the OFC and dACC could be linked to adjustments of own confidence after flawed judgements or errors, particularly when no external feedback was provided; hinting at control mechanisms to assess the own accuracy of self-judgements. It is notable, that there is a difference between external feedback and no external feedback, which hints at different mechanisms at play, when one's flaws can be seen (and judged) by others, against instances where this is not the case. In other words: it is easier to admit a flaw, error or shortcoming before oneself privately than before others; an important cue in social comparison contexts. The *ventral Anterior Cingulate Cortex* is another region important for social evaluation processes, as it has been established, that its primary activation happens in identifying the valence (whether positive or negative) of personality traits. While it does not appear to predict individual differences in upward comparison, it is more involved in processing rewarding vs. non-rewarding traits (Beer & Hughes, 2009).

Lastly, Kedia et al. (2014) mention, that the dACC is also activated during social comparison processes, that reult in envy, when others are perceived as superior. Similarly, the lateral part of the OFC is active during the processing of negative evaluation outcomes and pubishments, i. e. feeling inferior. Several studies support the conclusions, that there are specifically the dACC and the OFC in heightened activity, when social comparisons yield unfavorable results for the self. For instance, Takahashi et al. (2009) used fMRI investigations to prove, that when participants reported feelings of envy, they exhibited increased activity in the dACC, making it a key region for the negative outcomes in social comparison. Furthermore, the feeling of 'schadenfreude', which describes negative outcomes for the perceived *superior* individuals could be linked to increased activity in the ventral striatum – as a part of the brain's reward system, it suggests, that individuals in social comparison settings feel similarly 'rewarded' by negative outcomes for superior humans as when they receive own rewards; the reflected feeling is derived from the German language: *schadenfreude: 'Schaden'* translating to *damage* and *'Freude'* meaning *pleasure.* Additionally, the study was able to show, that the degree of activity in the dACC region when reporting feelings of envy could predict the degree of ventral stratial activity in experiencing schadenfreude accordingly.

In 2007, Fliessbach et al. had found evidence for modulation in the ventral striatum in response to relative rewards – the pleasure of reward depended on whether peers were rewarded more or less in comparison. Accordingly, the lateral region of the OFC could be found in increased activity when rewarded, but less than others, aligning with feelings of inferiority and dissatisfaction. This is particularly interesting because reward appears to be highly relative in the context of social comparison; it does not necessarily evoke positive associations, since it must be perceived relative to peers and can even trigger negative evaluations, proven by according brain activity. The schematic activity map below provides insight in important activations of the aforementioned regions in the discussed social scenarios:

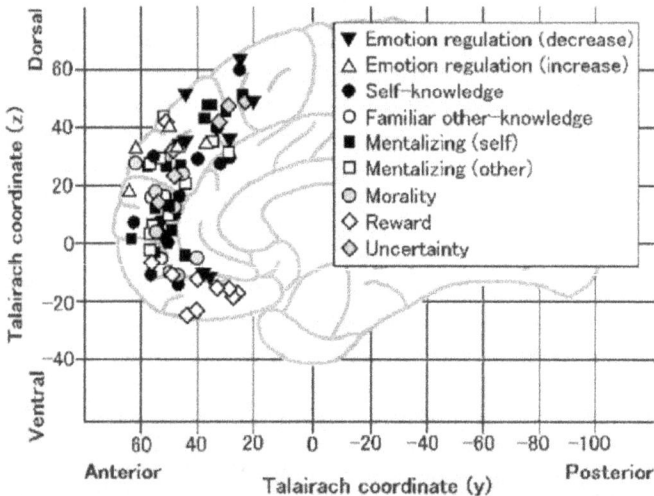

Figure 2: Schematic Mapping of the Medial Prefrontal Cortex activations in response to social settings, compiled by Nakao et al. (2009) according to their literature review.

Moreover, a 2016 study led by Kumaran et al. could reveal specific activity in the Medial Prefrontal Cortex in subjects when they updated their knowledge on social status; the study compared the mPFC region activity in social hierarchy learning with other information and could establish, that during the process of updating objective measures of social hierarchy information in the self, the activity in the mPFC region significantly increased. The below figure is taken from their study *Computations Underlying Social Hierarchy Learning: Distinct Neural Mechanisms for Updating and Representing Self-Relevant Information.*

Derived from that, and in alignment with the previous findings by Nakao et al., we can establish, that social comparison with other individuals triggers certain activity in defined brain regions in relation to self-assessment. That is, it

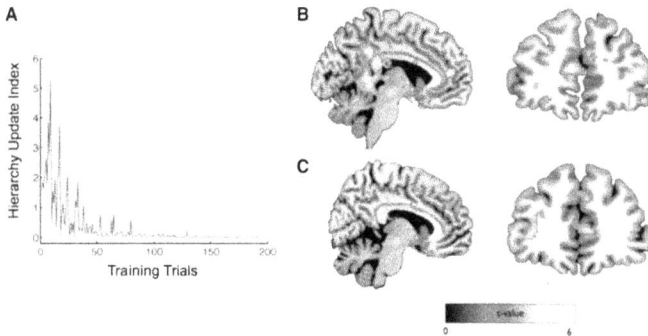

Figure 3: Kumaran et al. (2016): It is clearly visible how in (B) there shows a significant correlation between heightened activity in the mPFC region in question and the update process in social hierarchy information, in comparison to (C), which represents 'other condition'.

can be perceived as a genetic trait, that we show a biological response to social comparison in very specific ways, which solidified the importance of upward and downward comparisons for our social identity; not only in a psychological, but also a neurobiological manner. Equipped with supporting evidence, it becomes clear how we are intrinsically wired to perform social comparison for our identity evolution, which leads us to the assumption, that significant changes in the social environments we find ourselves in (i. e. the advent of social media with the prevailing large-scale idealization) will also have significant effects on how our brains process these new arrays of social information.

Contemporary research conducted by Dwortz et al. (2022) proposes, that there is an evolutionary element in processing social hierarchies and status signals, with involvement of certain brain regions. The figure below shows a schematic illustration.

After we have now understood more about the cognitive mechanisms in social comparison, our next question to clarify would be the changes and adaptations in frequency, in which social comparison happens in modern digital times. Research

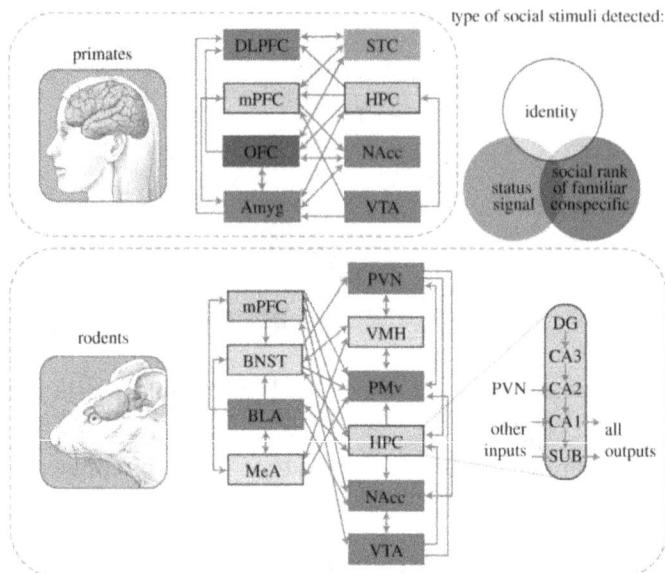

Figure 4: Brain systems involved in the representation of a dominance hierarchy; grey lines representing anatomical connectivity across regions; Dorsolateral Prefrontal Cortex (DLPFC), Medial Prefrontal Cortex (mPFC), Orbitofrontal Cortex (OFC), Amygdala (Amyg), Superior Temporal Cortex (STC), Hippocampus (HPC), Nucleus Accumbens (NAcc), Ventral Tegmental Area (VTA) – Figure by Dwortz et al. (2022).

providing answers to this specific question appears to be still limited; however, there are a number of works, that provide deeper insight into the dynamics, that the omnipresence of digital networks brings forth. Pellegrino (2024) found, that it is especially the algorithmic bias, that drives intense upward comparisons, because it displays the most liked content most frequently and prominently. From what we have established so far, the relatively new digital social metrics can be perceived as status symbols of their own, which could be an important factor in our assessment. Since those who appear most socially desirable are becoming increasingly prevalent in social media, it would be only natural, that more individuals compare themselves to their exhibited personality traits and aspire to align with them. Public visibility of their real-time social standing, measured in likes, follower numbers and similar could be convincing arguments for individuals to frequently compare their own lives with the displayed personas. As we will later learn, cognitive reinforcement is a strong force at play in the dynamics of algorithmic curation of content, and it can be strongly linked to the compulsion with which many users act in digital environments nowadays. Ling et al. (2023) found links between age ranges and the susceptibility to the displayed idealization, explaining that in general, younger audiences are more likely to be heavily influenced; especially in evoking materialistic attitudes, feelings of envy and inadequacy. Franz (2014) could establish, that there are stronger emotional effects in users, who can be seen as susceptible to overly frequent social comparison in the first place. After all, Midgley (2013), Foddy & Crundall (1993), and Wilson & Ross (2000) suggest, that social comparison, and upward comparison in particular do indeed have become more frequent, albeit some of the works identified reasons other than social media, e. g. changing conditions in workplaces and increased competitiveness – given their publication time prior to social media's advent, that is natural, and it also makes the observations more complete as to be able to identify diverse reasons for the general increase in these behaviors. However, as we will be able to solidify at a later point, it is especially the rise of new forms of reinforcement loops, that have further exacerbated the compulsive element in those behaviors. At this point, we have set the stage for our next theme complex: a scientific assessment of the consequences these dynamic societal shifts have, by careful subsumption of the psychological impact of amplified social validation needs under Alfred Adler's famous theory of the *Inferiority Complex*.

4.3 Alfred Adler's Inferiority Complex: A Psychological Basis for Social Comparison

Alfred Adler's concept of the inferiority complex serves as a fundamental element in understanding the psychological foundations of social comparison. His pioneering work in individual psychology suggests, that human beings are intrinsically driven by a feeling of inferiority, which they seek to diminish. In Adler's opinion, this sense of being inferior to others originates from early childhood experiences, that are naturally characterized by helplessness, vulnerability and dependence (Adler, 1927/1997). As one of the fundamental aspects of Adler's psychological framework, he posited that the perceived inferiority propel individuals to a natural pursuit of its very opposite; superiority. Importantly, this must not be misunderstood as an inherent desire for dominance, as in a negative or oppressive manner; rather, the human nature of striving to achieve superiority, according to Adler (1956/1964), is a constant and ongoing commitment to self-improvement and overcoming life's obstacles. Viewed through this perspective, it shows how feelings of inferiority and inadequacy are sought to be compensated and how they may link to obtaining social validation.

According to Adler (1929/2013), these feelings of inferiority are not inherently detrimental; he emphasized how they can serve as a strong catalyst for personal growth and development, resulting in positive contributions to society – given they are managed properly. One of the central themes in Adler's interpretations is the proper management of one's perceived inferiority, which he believed are a natural and necessary part of growing up. Difficulties arise, however, when the feelings of inadequacy become overwhelming, so that they impair one's proper functioning – this condition, deemed *Inferiority Complex*, is an important pillar of his research and therapy efforts and has shaped psychology and philosophy significantly (Adler, 1933/2009). As opposed to general feelings of inferiority, the inferiority complex does indeed bring significant detriment for the patient, and thus is to be strictly distinguished. The reason why Adler's psychological framework is an essential cornerstone of this book becomes clear in a particular work by Adler (1931/2011), suggesting that the aforementioned condition is often exacerbated by a constant tendency to compulsively compare oneself with others, especially in settings where social status, achievement and personal values are continually evaluated against external standards. Little could Adler know at the time how deep mankind would spiral into the abyss of inferiority over the course of a century.

As one of his core findings, Adler (1927/1997) articulated, that every individual enters life in a state of complete dependence, relying solely on others for their well-being. According to him, the experienced state of reliance fosters a natural sense of inferiority, because children recognize and internalize the disparity between their own capabilities, knowledge and autonomy and that of adults or older peers. In his opinion, the consciousness of being smaller, weaker and generally less capable than others is a source of inspiration for children. It sparks their wish to achieve greater competence, mastery and independence. Adler (1925) argued that the feeling of inferiority is not limited to physical attributed like bodily strength or height, but also extends to psychological dimensions, as children begin to compare themselves with their peers in proximate social surroundings. As they observe their skills, knowledge or social standing they may experience how they fall short, upon which they form goals and individual aspirations. According to Adler, this process reflects how individuals are prompted to seek ways to transcend their individually perceived limitations and live up to their surroundings. Adler termed this process the '*compensatory* striving for superiority' – serving as a motivator born from the experience of being inferior. In his work *Problems of Neurosis* (1929/1999), he asserted that inferiority is an unavoidable aspect of life, and expands from childhood throughout adult life: as individuals have to navigate through ever new challenges, irrespective of their maturity state, they face social relationships and societal expectations, where they seek to establish an own sense of competence. Challenges, however, be they physical, intellectual or emotional, arise at every stage of life, letting individuals of all ages encounter occasional feelings of inferiority in relation to others who are perceived as more accomplished, respectively. Adler (1933/2009) perceived this dynamic as an essential part of personal growth, as one's identity is substantially shaped by the inherent drive to overcome challenges, at whose core must be the own realization and acknowledgement of individual limitations.

Adler made an important distinction between natural feelings of inferiority, as described above, and the pathological condition known as the inferiority complex. As opposed to the former, where individuals experience the natural occurence of inferiority in a healthy manner and steer their feelings toward personal growth, the pathological condition repesents a maladaptive response to these feelings. According to Adler (1933/2009), natural feelings of inferiority are typically temporary and should ideally have a motivating effect. In contrast, the inferiority complex is deeply ingrained and has a paralyzing effect. The paralysis causes the individual to obsessively ponder their perceived shortcomings and develop a strong fixation on self-doubt. Consequently, the feeling of inadequacy does *not* lead to motivation and overcoming challenges, but becomes a persistent and negative condition, where one's natural shortcomings are perceived irrationally and exaggeratedly (Adler, 1931/2011). As other scholars have pointed out, the distortion of reality that results from these irrational perceptions, can result in exaggerated efforts to protect the self-esteem, for instance through the development of unrealistic expectations for oneself or others, further exacerbating the continual feeling of failure and disappointment (Mosak & Maniacci, 1999) – consequently, the inferiority complex results in the very opposite of healthily processed feelings of inferiority. It inhibits personal growth and confines individuals in a cycle of self-defeat (Feist & Feist, 2008).

Moreover, Watts (2013) and Gilbert (2016) have further elaborated on Adler's theories, with their works highlighting an important point that joints the original thoughts with modern era societal dynamics: they emphasize, that growing social pressures and the general expectation of performance and achievement foster an environment of perpetual competition. These strong external amplifications can be seen as particular fuel for the prevailing inferiority complex, strengthening the own ill-sitting beliefs of irrational inferiority and entrenching the sense of inadequacy and failure. While Adler (1927) stated, that formative years are especially influential in the development of identity and coping with inferiority, the amount and quality of validation provided by caregivers is a critical cornerstone in the mechanisms an individual will develop for their future management of inferior feelings. A significant lack of approval or repeated failure without corrective feedback and instruction may solidify feelings of inadequacy that can persist lifelong; through this influence in later behavior, individuals develop tendencies to continuously compare themselves to others, in order to validate their self-worth. This dynamic is particularly interesting in light of the perpetuated realization of inadequacy that it carries – as we have established, the distortion of reality and rationality in expectations, in unison with compulsive comparisons, can end in a tremendous spiral of experienced inferiority, to an extent where it significantly diminishes self-worth. In contrast, he posits that early encouragement and positive social feedback helps prevent the reinforcement of inferiority in an unhealthy manner and rather fosters healthy coping mechanisms through the experience, that failure and inferiority are natural, yet can be overcome. In addition, this means, that healthy intervention may function as an educative factor in developing rational expectations. In later works and modern individual psychology with numerous different influences, Sweeney (1998) describes, how specifically avoidance behavior is tackled, so that individuals develop a sense of resilience and are enabled to perceive inferiority as a motivator, which reestablishes healthies coping mechanisms and also strive for self-improvement instead of compulsive self-defeat.

As a consequence to what has been clarified above, it becomes evident, that in shaping one's identity, there is a delicate balance between inferiority and superiority and the healthy processing of each, especially in light of the pathological conditions in perceiving oneself as inferior to others, and the applied doping mechanisms, that the individual may not even be aware of. Alfred Alder (1927) describes, how one of the key characteristics of an inferiority complex is that the individual attempts to conceal their according insecurities and inadequacy through overcompensation. According to Horney (1973), this overcompensation typically manifests in a relentless pursuit of dominance (as we may recall at this point, Adler himself described healthy pursuit of *superiority* as explicitly not equal with seeking particular *dominance*), often accompanied with outward aggression and the compulsive need for success. This happens in an attempt to mask inner feelings of inferiority and insecurity, which are not healthily processed, and which, at that point, have already manifested in a detrimental manner. The inferiority is no more any source of inspiration, but has become a painful realization of diminished worth and has a toxic effect on cognition and behavior. Kernberg (1975) went further and described how this drive can get out of control for the individual, when the inferiority and its subsequent overcompensation reach a state that is unmanageable. In those instances, there is a possibility, that grandiosity and the compulsive showcasing of superiority culminate in excessive need for validation, at the cost of positive character traits, i.e. the development of narcissistic tendencies. At this point, concealing the inner insecurity is the most important driver for behavior, and the low self-esteem leads to not only overcompensation in the personal pursuit of superiority but also in the active denigration and belittling of others to maintain a sense of superiority. Thus, when overcompensation evolves into narcissism, the damage shifts from being largely inward, affecting the individual's own sense of self, to being outwardly destructive, affecting the individual's relationships and environments. Narcissistic behavior, in this regard, is not merely about self-enhancement but also about undermining the value of others. Adler himself (1929) noted, how he observed pathological aggression in response to perceived threats from the outside – which can be seen as a pre-stage of the aforementioned escalation into pathological narcissism. The ongoing need to assert superiority in order to cope with the inner conflict of feeling inferior displayed in hostility and overdriven defensiveness, most certainly in an attempt to prevent one's deeply hidden inadequacy from being revealed. Expanding on the exhibited aggression, Vaillant (1993) notes impulsivity in the engagement of reckless and harmful behaviors in both encapsulating own poor self-assessment as an inward self-defensive mechanism and in attempts to outwardly reflect and demonstrate value.

Carl G. Jung (1954) on the other hand described how individuals might choose less outwardly damaging or even destructive ways to avoid revelation of their hidden flaws, in largely withdrawing from social situations. The intention behind seeking isolation however was the same, according to Jung; concealing imperfection as a response to ill-sitting self-assessments and irrationally processed feelings of inferiority. As we have previously established, the tendency to raise one's own standards and develop irrational expectations and demands from the self can lead to what Blatt (1995) calls *maladaptive perfectionism*. The constant striving for flawlessness with self-set unrealistic life standards, which are based upon unmanaged feelings of inferiority that have gotten out of manageable control, can lead to a spiral of failing attempts of compensation with the perpetuated reinforcement of feelings of inadequacy, failure, and as Blatt (1995) states – *depression*. Blatt's work will prove to be a significant cornerstone in weaving several of the loose ties together in the realm of this book; hence we will return to his publication *The Destructiveness of Perfectionism: Implications for the Treatment of Depression* at a later time. In more severe cases, where there seems to be a limitation to what can be achieved through relentless perfectionism, individuals have exhibited rather severe distortions of their reality and adjustment of facts to match their own perception (Rogers, 1951), which also provides a clear insight in how the self-defense mechanism of overcompensation may even lead to fabrication of false success stories to mask perceived failures. This aligns with Rogers's sophisticated explanations of how individuals do even organize organic experiences into their framework of self. Rogers describes a disjointed conscious perception and organic perception, with the only consciously perceived feelings being those, that can be brought into alignment with the own concept of the self, whilst distorting others to a degree that matches the self-concept. What Rogers describes as 'denial' can reach fascinating extents, according to his well-documented cases:

> It should be noted that perceptions are excluded because they are contradictory, not because they are derogatory. It seems nearly as difficult to accept a perception which would alter the self-concept in an expanding or socially acceptable direction as to accept an experience which would alter it in a constricting or socially disapproved direction. The self-distrusting client cited above has as much difficulty accepting her intelligence as a person with a self-concept of superiority would have in accepting experiences indicating mediocrity. Many perplexing issues are connected with the question, How is the denial effected? As we studies our clinical material and recorded cases, some of us – including the writer – began to develop the theory that in some way an experience could be recognized as threatening and prevented from entering awareness, without the person ever having been conscious of it, even momentarily. (p. 506).

Rogers's accounts are a strong indicator of how the internalized self-concept in cases of pathological inferiority is an extraordinarily strong force in identity development (albeit not in terms of a classic inferiority complex, but still noteworthy at this point), and how deep the own perceptions of inferiority can sit; it is intriguing how the patient's concept of her own self could be characterized by such low self-esteem that she was unable to integrate an acceptance of her own intelligence in her self-assessment. In my opinion, the described extent to which denial can distort the self-perception is a weighty argument for both, how a reinforced sense of inferiority can shape personality deeply and also how it can become the driving force in one's overcompensation, up ton the point where objective reality is negated.

According to Millon (1996), the own inner pressure of overcompensation can lead to fluctuations between inflated self-perception and low self-worth, which underlines the shifts that individuals go through when they feel the societal pressure of keeping up with what they seek to reflect and experiencing the self-made dichotomy between their presented persona and what they feel about their own inadequacy. This cycle may be reminiscent of one of the core theories presented in this books unified perspective in the beginning: amplitudinal cycling between rushes of positive validation followed by realization of the intrinsic shallowness of this very pursuit. Furthermore, it is only natural, how the frequent oscillations in behavior, coupled with outwardly aggressive defense can strain interpersonal repationships. In the false belief, that others are willing to expose one's weaknesses and the perceived inferiority that they attempt to conceal, conflicts arise. This can lead to alienation of social connections and complicate the maintenance of healthy relationships (Beck, 1990).

Pathological compensation, as noted by Freud (1936), is characterized by an individual's difficulty to accept vulnerability. This often results in a continuous pursuit of power, i.e. dominance, and the constant need for external validation. In their efforts to address their internal emotional void, individuals frequently resort to the only coping mechanisms they are familiar with. The vulnerable inner self, which has experienced significant emotional strain, must be protected at all costs. The underlying conflicts driving such behaviors, as indicated through the analysis of Adler's works, stem from a recognition of inferiority, which must be concealed from others. This internal struggle can lead to aggressive defensive behavior and a pathological denial of one's feelings, inhibiting acceptance. Consequently, clinical interventions must first cultivate an understanding of the origins of these behaviors before they can effectively address them. Ellis (1962) advocates for cognitive-behavioral approaches to target the pathological manifestations of inferiority and to introduce healthier coping mechanisms gradually. This process involves adjusting the distorted sense of self that has evolved over time, which often includes a reluctance to acknowledge personal flaws and an accumulation of overcompensation (as seen in Rogers's case documentations). Through an unrelenting pursuit of negative superiority, individuals not only alienate those around them but also drift ever further from recognizing and accepting that failure is a natural component of life, and that feelings of inferiority need not be excessively compensated for.

4.4 Social Manifestations of Psychopathological Inferiority

In order to integrate pathological inferiority with the influences modern social dynamics, it is worth working through its numerous effects in social behavior. As mentioned before, the long-term manifestation of negatively processed inferiority causes the individual to develop a strong focus on their perceived inadequacy, which can lead to substantial social withdrawal and a manifestation of avoidance patterns. Albeit often heavily distorted, the perceived reality invokes a gripping fear of judgment and exposition (Gilbert & Irons, 2009; Strano & Petrocelli, 2005), which can make social isolation the only 'safe haven' in order to not be confronted with one's own shortcomings or failure. This all is an attempt to avoid what is felt as exposing oneself to 'social risks', because even normal social encounters that do not bear the probability of strong judgment are increasingly perceived as threatening to one's own safe space (Alden & Taylor, 2004; Heimberg et al., 2010), which results in isolation to prevent further validation and reinforcement of inferiority. What we can derive from this is that the excruciating pressure and strain felt from the own *focus* on flaws is capable of distorting an individual's reality in such a way, that the own focus is *projected* outwardly; the readiness for defense and the will to hide insecurities is so strong, that there is a certainty that others will focus on the very flaw as well. This pathology can be compared to relatively newly discovered *Body Dysmorphic Disorder* (BDD), where individuals possess a minor bodily flaw, on which they project their entire focus spending considerable mounts of time to conceal it, withdraw socially and experience a debilitating pressure stemming from the belief that others are constantly focusing on their flaw, albeit it would not be regarded as abnormal or even noticeable by others (JefferiesSewell et al., 2016). Describing the condition, Jefferies-Sewell et al. quote contributing knowledge when they argue, that individuals fear showing their 'imperfection' publicly (Rosen, 1995) which leads to social avoidance patterns and isolation (Goodman et al., 1989) whilst troubling over a minor bodily imperfection that is often unnoticed by others (Grant & Phillips, 2005). Consequently, the internal focus causes *hypervigilance*, characterized by constant monitoring of cues for others' opinions, leading to immense pressure and further validating the need for compulsively hiding and concealing the inadequacy (Clark & Wells, 1995). On the other hand, one of the behavioral patterns which will be particularly important in light of excess modern social validation is the heightened need for external approval, as described by Mongrain (1998), who argues, that distress-causing feelings of inferiority can drive inhealthy needs for social approval as a compensating counterweight, which may result in generally unhealthy social behaviors. External approval and general social comparison often correlate, especially in the context of modern media, where newly introduced metrics make social validation measurable for the individual and the public likewise. As Mussweiler et al. (2004) argued, the comparisons mainly result in negative assessments, which further entrenches and validates the own inadequacy, most adding to the negative spiral instead of fostering own motivation and well-being. Moreover, Beck at al. (1985) highlight the cognitive bias with which those individuals approach social interactions, underscoring the inevitable negative assessment of each social encounter, because social interactions are interpreted with such high individual bias that the inferior self-perception functions like a self-fulfilling prophecy. Conclusively, the pathological inferiority is a vicious cycle, as it diminishes self-worth considerably, while at the same time strengthens the belief in it, having individuals engage in exactly those sort of behaviors that reinforce the truthfulness and the apparent alignment with others' image of oneself. A self-powering machine, which, unless careful intervention breaks it, likely goes on infinitely.

In a recent study, Zhao et al. (2024) highlighted, that public personas on social networks typically post the positive aspects of their lives, including symbols of status and wealth and explicitly highlighting the socially desirable sides of life and their curated personas. This phenomenon has been assessed before, and it is an important factor in the consideration how modern digital media influences individuals in their self-assessment. In being constantly reminded of others' achievements, including the aspects that may be 'better' in their lives, it is natural that they invoke feelings of inferiority when comparing one's own life with these unattainable standards.

Through the digital 'currency' of likes and comments etc., that nowadays measure social value, the social status becomes directly comparable and scalable in comparison to others, which is something that previous eras lacked. It is not only the visual impression of how beautiful and successful others are, it is the direct comparability and scalability to one's own 'miserable' status, that entrenches the superiority they showcase, and reinforces the deep-sitting inferiority in viewers. While the personas are carefully idealized to closely resemble societal ideals (Yang & Brown, 2016), social comparison becomes an inevitable disappointment. The only logical conclusion in comparing the unrealistic life standards other appear to have, and one's own – which are, of course, unfiltered to the self – must end up in the conclusion, that oneself is living a life that is inferior in almost any aspect. Thus, the constant exposure to modern forms of social representation plays a significant role in the reinforcement of inferiority; while there is no reason to believe, that the effects and consequences would be any different from what we have established above.

Especial attention should be given to instances, where there is a prevailing inferiority complex that has already pathological character: in prevalent online environments characterized by perpetual social competition, the chances of solidifying inner dissatisfaction and inferiority are significant, while positive contributions are neglegible. As social comparison has significantly escalated in contemporary online dynamics, the assumption that the inferiority complex is more relevant than ever is logical. As we are walking down the avenue of relying increasingly on digital self-promotion, for leisure and professional purposes, self-perception and confidence can take significant blows by the constant confrontation with individuals that seem to do everything better than ourselves. However, paired with a prevailing pathological inferiority complex, the consequences can be dramatically exacerbated through the permanent fuel that is added in ways

Adler could hardly have anticipated in his contemporary explanations. At this point, I would like to revisit Blatt (1995), who shared his concept of the emotional and cognitive toxicity of perfectionism, which blends into the vicious and self-perpetuating cycle. The internalized feelings of inferiority are met by mitigating attempts characterized by setting impractically high standards for themselves. Blatt emphasizes the detrimental effects of this perfectionism tendencies, particularly when the self-set standards are not met. Consequences can be emotional stagnation and cycles of self-criticism further diminishing one's self-image. However, there is also 'socially prescribed' perfectionism, aligning with the continuous display of questionable perfection in online environments: as an intensifying factor, social media amplifies the associated anxiety and fear of social rejection, culminating in a cyclical trap of relentlessly pursuing (and failing) perfection. As we now know, these perceived failures do even further increase the compulsivity with which individuals seek validation (and fail again), and also compare themselves to ('perfect') others. This loop can only end in emotionally debilitating feelings of worthlessness and total failure, sustaining a spiral of anxiety and emotional distress.

5 The Neurochemical Foundations of Social Validation in Modern Contexts

To avoid that this section becomes overly dense and exhausting, I will follow a strict framework to govern my elaborations. Addressing the neurochemical dynamics is a crucial component of shedding light on how modern dynamics in digital environments lead individuals to the widely observed behavioral patterns we can see today, accompanied by the psychological detriment, that might go as far as define new mental health conditions and illnesses based on the fast developments we experience these days. Having conducted research in different settings of secondary education for several years, documenting relevant observations and still being actively involved in adult professional rehabilitation, I am now more than ever convinced, that over the course of the next years and decades, we will be in need of refining existing knowledge on mental illnesses and we will also witness the emergence of ones original to digital natives, hence that will be grounded in, and derived from our modern world and way of life. It is specifically the relentlessness of mentally taxing dynamics our modern society exhibits, that leads to the similarity in psychological suffering in an exponentially growing number of individuals. Thus, the framework I will follow shall balance accessibility with the necessary rigor and depth and is intended to cover the following focal points:

- The brain's reward system, more specifically

  - *Ventral Tegmental Area (VTA)*
  - *Nucleus Accumbens*
  - *Prefrontal Cortex (PFC)*
  - *Dorsal and Ventral Striatum*
  - *Anterior Cingulate Cortex*
  - *Orbitofrontal Cortex*
  - *Amygdala*
  - *Hippocampus*

- The concept of cognitive reinforcement, specifically variable reinforcement schedules as seen in operand conditioning

- Dopamine release in response to social stimuli (i.e. reward anticipation and reception)

- The balance of dopamine and serotonin, *as far as we understand it today*

- The influence of this oscillation on the dopamine-serotonin interaction and consequently on well-being.

5.1 A Brief Introduction to the Brain's Reward System

The following anatomical figure provides an overview of the locations of important regions involved in reward processing, and which will be distinctly explained according to their relevant role for our perspective below.

5.1.1 Ventral Tegmental Area

The Ventral Tegmental Area (VTA) is located in the midbrain (Schultz 1998; Schultz, 2015). Besides containing glutamate and GABA neurons, it mainly contains dopamine neurons

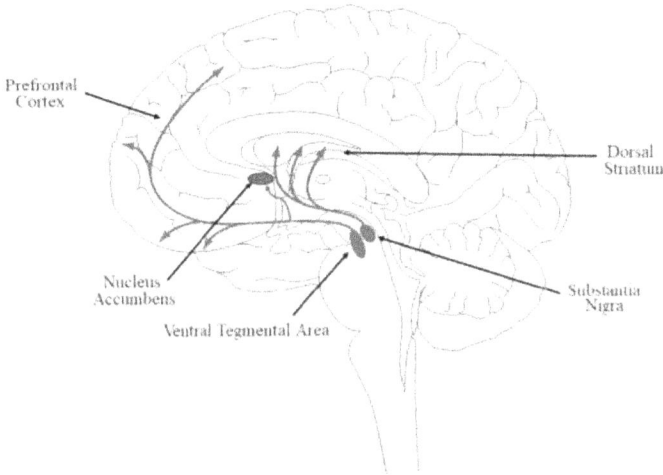

Figure 5: Dopamine System, Map from Morales & Barbano (2023).

and thus plays a central role in the mediation of dopamine release and thus the functions that are linked to the release of dopamine. Dopamine is a neurotransmitter that is crucial for motivation and processing rewards (Cai & Tong, 2022), we will elaborate on its specifics in more detail at a later point. According to Khayat & Yaka (2024), Bouarab et al. (2019) and Koutlas et al. (2024), dopaminergic neurons in the VTA activate during the anticipation of reward reception, thus reinforcing behaviors that are linked to reward-seeking. While Palmer et al. (2024) explain a strong influence of the VTA's dopaminergic output on the *Nucleus Accumbens*, which is central to the evaluation of rewards and plays an important role in addiction, Yalçin et al. (2024) found myelin plasticity in the VTA's neurons, which is an important indicator of adaptability in this region. Furthermore, the VTA is connected to motor regions in the brain, which might suggest a connectivity between reward anticipation feedback loops and physical actions (Astrakas et al., 2023).

5.1.2 Nucleus Accumbens

The Nucleus Accumbens (NAc) mediates and integrates signals of reward and motivation through inputs from the VTA. Through that, it is crucial for the reinforcement of rewarding behavior: GABA, or gamma-aminobutyric acid, is an inhibitory neurotransmitter, and these GABAergic projections work by inhibiting cholinergic interneurons in the NAc. Cholinergic interneurons are responsible for modulating the excitatory neurotransmission that influences reward processing in the brain. By inhibiting these cholinergic interneurons, the GABAergic projections from the VTA reduce their activity, thereby influencing the overall reward-related signaling in the NAc. This inhibitory control can decrease the activity of pathways that promote reward-seeking behavior, effectively regulating how the brain responds to rewarding stimuli. Al-Hasani et al. (2021) suggest that this mechanism is an important aspect of the brain's ability to balance reward behavior, helping to fine-tune the response to rewards and potentially avoid maladaptive behaviors like addiction, which we will later highlight is a crucial aspect in assessing the reward system and reinforcement of behavior. Importantly, the NAc received input from other important involved regions, among which particularly the *Amygdala* and the *Prefrontal Cortex* are important for the memory and emotional and cognitive evaluation of rewards (Sesack & Grace, 2010). Zheng et al. (2007) further found, how the NAc and the VTA work together in processing dopamine pathways for rewards, both druginduced and natural. The NAc has been found to connect its medial spiny neurons back to nondopaminergic neurons in the VTA which can be described as a critical feedback loop for reward regulation (Xia et al., 2011).

5.1.3 Prefrontal Cortex

The Prefrontal Cortex (PFC), mainly involved in emotion regulation, insight and reponse flexibility, has an important role in the complex dopaminergic brain process. Firstly, PFC neurons are connected to both dopaminergic and GABAergic neurons in the VTA, which influences VTA's dopamine output to the PFC itself and the nucleus accumbens (Carr & Sesack, 2000). This is particularly interesting since it is a circuitry that is capable of influencing its own dopamine input and subsequent processing: PFC-VTA connectivity uses glutamatergic projections to the VTA, exciting dopaminergic neurons which project back to the PFC and the NAc; however, through GABAergic neurons responsible for the inhibition of dopaminergic ones, the PFC exhibits control over the regulation of dopaminergic neuron activity and output; thereby controlling its own dopamine input. In 1984, Dunnet et al. found, that stimulation of the PFC can trigger dopamine release in the NAc reinforcing the role of the PFC in reward-seeking behavior; however through factoring in the connectivity with inhibitory neurons in the VTA, the modulation of dopamine release links cognitive control with reward and subsequent emotional processing (Sesack & Pickel, 1992; Taber et al., 1995). The dynamic connectivity we know from other regions of the brain is important to be remembered at this point, since no part in this interplay is merely active or passive; all is dynamic. This is supported by findings, that could highlight, that inactivation of the VTA affects the synchronization between the PFC and the NAc, significantly impairing the intrinsic motivation for reward-related behavior in individuals (Cortes et al., 2019).

5.1.4 Dorsal and Ventral Striatum

The dorsal and ventral striatum are interconnected yet have distinct roles in the dopaminergic system. The dorsal striatum receives dopaminergic input from both the *Substantia Nigra* and the VTA and is primarily involved in motor control, which in this regard means its involvement in the regulation and formation of habitual behavior, or behavioral patterns (Zhang et al., 1997). The ventral striatum, of which the NAc is a part, is a key recipient of dopamine projections from the VTA, and is central to the processing of reward signals in learned behavior (Clarke & Adermark, 2015; Saberi, 2019). In interplay, they function as a unity in the formation of learning and habitualizing behavior that is linked to the reception of rewards. According to Albin (2019) and Humphries & Prescott (2010), learned behaviors transition from the ventral striatum to habis in the dorsal striatum, which highlights the importance of dopaminergic pathways for reinforcement learning. Generally, the VTA releases dopamine into both dorsal and ventral striatum, modulating motor control and behavioral learning (Keath et al., 2007). The NAc acts as an interface for the processing of rewards, and through interactions with the PFC, VTA and dorsal striatum, it helps to form habits (Park et al., 2019; Horvitz et al., 2002). Furthermore, the ventral striatum's connectivity with motor systems (dorsal s.) and also limbic systems (*Amygdala*) integrates cognitive and emotional inputs (Groenewegen et al., 2016; Haber, 2011).

I specifically like to quote Haber's (2011) excellent work *Neuroanatomy of Reward: A View from the Ventral Striatum*, since it has several profound implications for this section and well-beyond the ventral striatum subdivision. Her introduction alone is so well-executed that it serves as a highly valuable resource:

> [...] While the hypothalamus and other subcortical structures are involved in processing information about basic, or primary, rewards, higher-order cortical and subcortical forebrain structures are engaged when complex choices about these fundamental needs are required. [...] at the center of this network is the cortico-ventral basal ganglia (BG) circuit. This includes the orbitofrontal cortex (OFC) and anterior cingulate cortex (ACC), the ventral striatum (VS), the ventral pallidum (VP) and the midbrain dopamine (DA) neurons. [...] Other BG circuits, those associated with cognition and motor control, work in tandem with

elements of the reward system to develop appropriate goal-directed actions. [...] Moreover, the ventral striatal region receives a dense innervation from the amygdala, which is also tightly linked to sensory processing. [...] (Haber, 2011).

5.1.5 Anterior Cingulate Cortex

The Anterior Cingulate Cortex (ACC) has multiple connections with other critical brain areas in the dopaminergic circuitry, hence it plays an important role in balancing projections back and forth in the cycle of dopamine. It influences cost-benefit analyses in decision-making through dopaminergic signaling with dorsal and ventral striatum, in particular through integration of information from the dorsal striatum for further decision-making (Bolton et al., 2018; Assadi et al., 2019). Additionally, the ACC receives input projections from the VTA via dopamine pathways, accounting for its role in the regulation of reward prediction and goal-directed behavior, influencing both the PFC and the dorsal and ventral striatum (Bolton et al., 2018; Narita et al., 2010). The ACC integrates feedback via dopamine modulation, making it a key player in adapting behavior (Bush et al., 2000).

While the ACC interacts with circuits involving GABAergic neurons in the VTA and NAc modulating aversive behavior and balancing reward-seeking and aversive conditioning – its direct influence on these GABAergic circuits in the NAc is less established just yet (Zhou et al., 2022; Gao et al., 2020; Bush et al., 2000; Schweimer & Hauber, 2006; Al-Hasani, 2021). ACC inputs in the VTA may interact with glutamatergic neurons more directly than with GABAergic ones (Montardy et al., 2018). However, these dynamics prove crucial for the ACC's role in shaping adaptive responses to environmental stimuli.

5.1.6 Orbitofrontal Cortex

The Orbitofrontal Cortex (OFC), similarly to the PFC, is involved in the assessment of rewards, integrating dopaminergic inputs. Its primary role in the dopamine system is modulating decisions and reward-seeking based on the prediction and evaluation of outcomes (Del Arco & Mora, 2009; Groman et al., 2013; Takahashi et al., 2011; Wilson et al., 2014). Receiving dopmainergic inputs from tha VTA (Fitzgerald et al., 2009), it is responsible for comparative valuation, which could be described as the activity in reasoning if the reward is 'worth the effort'. Cetin et al. (2004) highlight its role in integrating dopamine input to assess and drive goal-directed behavior, which is a primary function for variable reinforcement schedules. Its role in the mesocortical pathway explains the regulation for social and agonistic behaviors (Bruin, 1990), shown in its behavior-regulating function through dopamine signaling, specifically in responses to social cues, processing their emotional and social significance (Bechara et al., Elliott & Deakin, 2005).

5.1.7 Amygdala

The amygdala's role in the human brain is primarily characterized by processing emotions, especially fear and aggression (Kienast et al., 2008), which it does by forming emotional memories. Through that function, it is responsible for aversion of threats and predicting dangers as negative outcomes (*'safety learning'*), but also learning and memory of tasks with emotional significance (Stubbendorff & Stevenson, 2021; Sagado-Pineda et al., 2005; Aksoy-Aksel et al., 2020). While it interacts with other brain regions not only through dopaminergic pathways, in the dopamine circuitry of the brain, it projects to the VTA, PFC, NAc and the hippocampus, utilizing dopaminergic pathways for emotional learning, anxiety regulation, stimulus-reward learning and consolidation of memories, as mentioned above (Kröner et al., 2005; Rossato et al., 2013; Fudge & Emiliano, 2003; Mc-

Gaugh, 2002; Hitchcott et al., 1997). Dopamine has been found to influence synaptic plasticity in the amygdala, emphasizing the adaptability with which emotional memories can be stored for learning and adaptation of behavior (Lee et al., 2017). Besides this, it is noteworthy, that the amygdala is also modulated by GABAergic neurons, so that there is a counterbalancing element that inhibits unrestricted dopamine in fear-related circuits to prevent overreacting to stimuli that might otherwise trigger intense, and perhaps uncontrollable fear responses; perhaps also in settings that would trigger social anxiety (Duvarci & Pare, 2014; Ehrlich et al., 2009).

5.1.8 Hippocampus

The hippocampus contains dopamine receptors which modulate synaptic plasticity and memory processing (Gangarossa et al., 2012; Tsetsenis et al., 2023), while dopamine plays an important role in long-term potentiation in the hippocampus, crucial for memory and learning (Baulac et al., 1986). The VTA projects to the hippocampus, regulating its excitability and influencing recognition memory in reponse to novel stimuli (Gasbarri et al., 1997; Titulaer, 2021). On the other hand, the hippocampus projects signals to other brain regions, such as the PFC and NAc, further involving it in cognitive processing and executive functions and also reward-learning (Thierry et al., 2000; Perez & Lodge, 2018). in 2005, Fujishiro et al. found, that dopamine interacts with acetylcholine (ACh) via the dopamine D2 receptors in the hippocampus, thereby affecting cognitive processes. Besides the Amygdala, the hippocampus is involved in aversive memory formation, since the hippocampus is especially sensitive to stress (Borgkvist et al., 2011; Tsetsenis et al., 2021).

5.2 The Principles of Cognitive Reinforcement

This part will delve into the principles of cognitive reinforcement, reinforcement learning and the foundations of variable reinforcement schedules, as they apply to the context of modern social dynamics, and especially to their neuropsychological underpinnings, in order to integrate them into the broader perspective. This is a means to shed some more light on why modern digital environments foster the behavioral patterns we can observe in large portions of society, and also examine the psychological effects they have. After all, through applying well-established principles in psychology alongside their neurochemical correspondents, the puzzle of how modern societal dynamics are well applicable pieces together more and more.

To introduce the basic concept of reinforcement, I would like to utilize the explanation I have shared in my previous work Cognitive Nemesis (2024):

> A fundamental concept in psychology and behavioral science, reinforcement, these days, is also one of the core mechanisms in deep learning, where machines use sophisticated algorithms to narrow down on a desired outcome and tailor their specifications to repetitive feedback. In cognitive and behavioral psychology, reinforcement, or reinforcement loops, refer to processes, in which certain behaviors, beliefs and convictions are strengthened through repetitive exposure to reinforcing stimuli. The principles of reinforcement can be seen as combinations of several observations in behavioral research over many decades. B. F. Skinner (1953) found, that shaping human behavior worked through carefully manipulating the consequences that follow it, eiher by positive reinforcement or by punishment. Through a form of posi-

tively experienced feedback, that is repeated, the likelihood of further exhibition of certain behavior increases. This is one of the seminal observations, that laid a foundation of behavioral science for decades to come. In 1972, Rescorla & Wagner found, that the processes that underly classical conditioning could be used to predict reinforcement processes. Through structured environments, human learning and decision-making could not only be heavily influenced, but also made predictable, to an extent. The concept of reinforcement could over time be extended through the social learning theory, introduced by Bandura (1977). Termed observational learning, individuals learned and reinforced certain behaviors by observing their peers, and mimicking their behaviors, which was an interesting finding, since it extended the understanding of reinforcement not through self-experienced consequences but also through others. In the context of this work, reinforcement as a concept is of high importance, because it is one of the fundamental mechanisms through which modern digital media is able to observe, predict and influence human behavior. [...] The scientific roots of these behavioral mechanisms can be traced back to seminal studies conducted by Skinner and Ivan Pavlov. Pavlov (1927) found, that through providing a certain stimulus (at the time, the behavior was trained on a dog), certain behavior could be reinforced. Pavlov termed this manipulation of behavior conditioning. Upon pairing the sound of a bell with food, upon which the dog salivated, the dog learned, that the bell was to be associated with food. Later on, the sound of the bell would be enough to evoke salivation. Skinner (1938) expanded on those principles by adding multiple factors of reinforcement or punishment, in order to not only solidify certain behaviors, but also eliminate others. These principles showed, how behavior could be manipulated through inherent experience, creating a whole new understanding of learning processes and the effects of consequence. The combination of those findings can be seen as the groundwork for a new understanding of learning and the possibilities to influence behavior. Modern age has its own adaptations of these fundamental principles in digital contexts, hence the understanding of the foundational principles is of such crucial importance. When we seek to understand, how and why observable behavioral phenomena in digital contexts are formed, it is essential to understand the basic mechanisms of human behavior and learning. (Gross, 2024, 9-11).

Before moving on, I would like to clarify, that reinforcement mechanisms are a critical part of the integrated perspective in this work, as they provide a fundamental understanding of how behaviors are shaped, maintained, and intensified through feedback mechanisms related to social validation and constant upward comparison. In the context of feelings of inferiority, contemporary social dynamics, and the brain's reward circuitry, the concept of reinforcement underlies many of the compulsive behaviors observed in today's society. Dopamine as a key component of the brain's reward system acts as a neurochemical reinforcer for behaviors that yield social approval, recognition, and achievement. As individuals pursue validation through social networks and other modern platforms, they engage in a continuous cycle of reinforcement. Positive feedback manifesting as likes, comments, or other forms of modern measurable praise – stimulates the brain's reward system, particularly areas such as the NAc and PFC, reinforcing the behavior and motivating individuals to seek additional validation. This results in a loop where individuals become increasingly reliant on external reinforcement to shape their self-esteem, prompting the recurrence of validation-seeking behaviors, often in a manner that can be described as compulsive. This momentum is closely linked to the characteristics of Adler's inferiority complex previously discussed, where individuals, feeling inadequate, turn to external validation to compensate for their perceived deficiencies, exhibiting increasingly compulsive behaviors to bear with their inner pressure. The unpredictable nature of social feedback, especially in digital contexts, resembles the variable reinforcement schedules explored by B.F. Skinner, which are known to strengthen behaviors and potentially lead to those compulsive behavior patterns, as they have been wellestablished to drive addiction. The interplay between neurochemical reinforcement, social comparison, and the constant feedback loop underscores the importance of reinforcement in understanding how modern social dynamics contribute to emotional and psychological instability, of which I propose the unnatural amplitudinal ups and downs in dopamine spikes and deficits may play a key role; on the one hand because they can be explained to deplete of serotonin and on the other hand because our brains are evidently not evolutionary equipped to handle such cyclical bursts of dopamine oscillations.

There are two distinct forms of reinforcement. The *negative*, where a negativ stimulus is removed as a consequence of desired behavior, which is bound to increase the frequency of desired behavior (Bandura, 1977), and the *positive*, where a positive stimulus is added when desired behavior occurs, reinforcing its frequency in occurence (Skinner, 1953). Primary reinforcers, such as food, warmth, and shelter, are innately rewarding and shape behavior without the need for prior learning (Hull, 1943). Evolution has played a critical role in creating the relevant linkages in both our behavior and brain structures that make us automatically recognize and seek these rewards for survival. This drive can be understood as an evolutionary adaptation, where survival depended on the ability to seek out and respond to vital resources. Without this automatic reinforcement mechanism, organisms might neglect essential behaviors, such as eating or finding warmth, which could result in starvation or death. Secondary reinforcers, which are learned behaviors, on the other hand, are not immediately essential for direct survival. Rewards like money or praise are those kind of rewards, that we have learned to associate with specific outcomes for ourselves (i.e. social standing, emotional well-being etc.), thereby having an indirect connection with primary reinforcers (Pavlov, 1927). As we have established earlier, it is indeed a crucial part of human evolution, that we seek social approval, yet it is not as directly associated with survival as food in the first place. However, especially in tribal age, it was social acceptance and the cohesion in the group, that ensured providing food and thus, there is the indirect connection between primary and secondary stilmuli. Premack (1965) found, that the better a consequence can be linked to a behavior, the better and the more effective the learning affect; in other words, the immediacy with which the consequence occurs upon a certain behavior, plays a vital role in the effectiveness of reinforcement. Schultz (1961), in accordance with variable reinforcement, found, that intermittent reinforcement patterns strengthen certain behavior over time, preventing extinction.

It is important to explain the two forms of *schedules* in reinforcement, as there are fixed and variable schedules that vary in their composition and effectiveness. According to Ferster & Skinner (1957), a fixed reinforcement schedule provides rewards after either a fixed number of responses or after a fixed amount of time. This means, that for the subject (i.e.: the *learner* of behavior), the reward becomes predictable. In terms of our analysis of the involved brain regions, there is the possibility of assessment; as we have established, it is specifically the orbitofrontal cortex, that receives dopaminergic input from the ventral tegmental area in order to reason between effort and reward value. On the other hand, variable reward schedules are classified into variable-ratio and variable-interval schedules. Variable-ratio reinforcement describes distribution of a reward after an unpredictable number of responses, which means, that for the individual, the state of expectancy is held at a high rate, because of its unpredictable nature. Any response to a stimulus could be the one yielding the next reward (Ferster & Skinner, 1957); while variable-interval schedules are based on the variablity in time intervals (Catania & Reynolds, 1968). Zeiler (1968), in accordance with previous findings, confirmed, that variable reinforcement is the most effective, because due to the unpredictable nature in reinforcement, it maintains a consistency in responses, thus yielding high rates of desired behavior. In addition, Ferster & Skinner (1957) proved, that variable-ratio reinforcement yields high *and* steady response rates. Translated to behavioral patterns, it can be concluded, that if not only a reward is linked to a behavior, but it is also unpredictable in nature, so as to remain in a state of hoping for a positive reward upon a response to a stimulus, it effectively reinforces behavior and creates a pattern. Additionally, it was found to produce consistently high engagement in reponses, as opposed to fixed reinforcement, which rather created 'pauses' (Catania, 1973). This might be on account of the predictability, that takes away the element of surprise and anticipation, leading to a state of saturation in satisfaction. While the rational element is triggered, when a reward can be anticipated, it does rather resemble compensation in exchange for 'work', while the element of unpredictability rises the nature of discovery and uncertainty, which triggers the 'gambling' element; as described by Mazur (1986). One particular aspect is critical in understanding: in the assessment of these reinforcement schedules, the effectiveness is entirely irrespective of how *beneficial* the actual behavior is to the individual. In other words: harmful behavior can be reinforced just as effectively. In the integration of reinforcement principles in our broader perspective, this will obviously play a key role.

There are numerous relatively young scientific findings that enhance our understanding of dopamine's important role in reinforcement. Firstly, Goedhoop et al. (2023) found, that dopamine is released during both the anticipation of a reward, and the reception of it, however the release is higher during the anticipation phase than during the actual reward. Dopamine ramps up before actions are taken to obtain the actual reward, which is a strong indicator for its prominent role in motivating actions in a prephase. This aligns with findings from Grimm et al. (2021) and Korb et al. (2020) who found dopamine diminishing during receipt and consumption of the reward, and rather exhibiting short bursts, as opposed to prolonged heightened levels during its anticipation.

Before further exploration of the development of habits through reinforcement processes within dopamine pathways, I see it as essential to clarify that the brain does not operate with a purely abstract or self-aware perspective when prioritizing certain behaviors. The brain should not be viewed as a self-conscious entity making autonomous decisions for its own interests. Instead, it functions according to biological imperatives that influence thoughts, emotions, and actions. The establishment of habitual actions does not result not from the brain 'choosing' to repeat them, but from physical changes occurring in its neural circuits – specifically through neuroplasticity and long-term potentiation (LTP) in critical areas. These neural changes are prompted by the repeated release of dopamine, which strengthens synaptic connections and enhances neural communication. This biological reinforcement allows the brain to replicate behaviors that have previously resulted in rewards. It is important to emphasize that the prioritization of behaviors is not arbitrary or theoretical; it is derived from concrete biological mechanisms that evolve in response to consistent stimuli. Without these mechanisms, we would not observe the consistency and uniformity of habit formation across different individuals; perhaps we would even perceive randomness and opposing behavioral patterns. Therefore, surges in dopamine alone do not deliver a sufficient explanation for behavioral prioritization; there must be underlying physical process in the brain facilitating this formation. In this context, the brain as an organ does not function as a self-aware '*driver*' of behavior but rather as the '*vehicle*' shaped by biological processes. These processes do not always align with an individual's well-being, yet they follow a somewhat predictable pattern based on the reinforcement of rewarding behaviors. As we will discuss further, the mechanistic nature of the brain's reward system, driven by dopamine pathways and neural plasticity, emphasizes why certain behaviors become prioritized and ultimately habitual. This explanation shall serve as one of the first foundations in bridging the question *why repeated dopamine surges do eventually heighten rewardseeking behaviors*, from observing that dopamine does surge in anticipation of reward, and the eventual observation that reward-seeking is habitualized; as the scientific perspective asks for what lies in between.

In a 2007 study, Nomoto et al. found, that midbrain dopamine neurons respond more intensely to complex and unpredictable stimuli, which can serve as an explanation for a stronger effectiveness in variable reward schedules. This effect is further intensified by fluctuations in reward timing. In a study by Claassen et al. (2017) in Parkinson's patients with compulsive behaviors, blood flow in the mesocorticolimbic are increased during unpredictable dopamine agonist therapy, which suggests that irregular rewards amplify dopamine surges and reinforcement processes. A key element here is *reward prediction error*: this concept describes dopamine spikes that indicate unexpected outcomes. A study on mice, led by Harada et al. in 2021, demonstrated that those animals exhibiting compulsive reward-seeking behavior displayed elevated AMPA/NMDA ratios in the orbitofrontal-striatal circuits, which reflected an increased sensitivity to unpredictability (*α-amino-3hydroxy-5-methyl-4-isoxazolepropinoic acid (AMPA) receptors are ionotropic receptors mediating fast synaptic transmissions. When glutamate binds to AMPA receptors, they allow Na^+ ions to enter the neuron, leading to excitatory postsynaptic potential (EPSP). Thus, they are involved in short-term synaptic plasticity. N-methyl-D-aspartate (NMDA) receptors on the other hand require both glutamate binding and postsynaptic depolarization to be activated. They allow the entry of Na^+ and Ca^{2+} ions to enter the neuron.*

While the influx of calcium is essential to trigger long-term potentiation (LTP), which is critical for learning and memory, NMDA receptors play a key role in long-term synaptic plasticity and neuroplasticity processes. The AMPA/NMDA ratio is often referred to as a metric in the investigation of synaptic strength and plasticity potential; a higher ratio indicates stronger connections between synapses and is therefore a marker for changes in synaptic activity, such as reward-seeking behavior, learning, memory and formation of habits (Purves et al., 2018; Hansen et al., 2018; Sheng et al., 2001; Traynelis et al., 2010).). Schultz (2002) explains prediction errors as a leraning tool that adjusts future expectations by recalibrating the brain's understanding of outcomes; through this mechanism dopamine release 'teaches' the brain how to fine-tune behaviors for future outcome maximization.

Seiler et al. (2022) were able to demonstrate how mice exhibited resistance to punishments while dopamine signaling in the dorsomedial striatum took place. This can be understood as a driving force in compulsion, even if punishment might await; it is critical in understanding, that rational assessment, from a certain point, is no longer part of compulsive behavior. Although conducted on mice, the study is an important argument for the dynamics of dopamine-driven compulsion. In 2010, Voon et al. found, that in individuals with compulsive gambling tendencies dopamine agonists intensified learning from gaining / winning experiences, with prediction error signals increasing and thereby strengthening compulsive behavioral patterns. Likewise, Harada et al. (2021) displayed, that enhanced dopamine signaling from orbitofrontal to striatal regions (in mice) heightened compulsive reward-seeking, *in particular* when rewards were inconsistently scheduled and thus unpredictable. Stuber et al. (2008) emphasize the strengthening of the brain's relevant circuitry hardwiring to favor similar actions. We remember at this point, how especially the striatum is a key brain region for learning and internalizing habitual behavior. In summary, these collective findings solidify that dopamine-driven responses to unpredictability in reward schedules significantly reinforce compulsive behavioral patterns under significant involvement of the striatum and the orbitofrontal cortex, and irrespective of rationality. Particularly the nucleus accumbens appears to play a critical role in the action initiation and motivation to act on the innate desire for rewards: Syed et al. (2015) highlight the increased dopamine release in the NAc as a driver for motivation upon dopamine surges, making it more likely for the individual to engage in further reward-seeking. This ties in the concept of positive reinforcement, as dopamine enhances the association between actions and reward-predicting cues (Pignatelli & Bonci, 2015). Lastly, as derived from research by Schultz (1998,2006) and Berridge & Robinson (1998), the difference deemed *'wanting* vs. *liking'*, very appropriately termed, describes the brain's differentiation between the feeling of pleasure during reward consumption (hedonic) and the motivational value to stimuli, representing the craving phase, in which dopamine plays a key role.

In the realm of this work and bridging back to modern social dynamics, one of the key aspects of reinforcement and dopamine's role in shaping behavior is compulsion. While certain behaviors emerge and can be observed, there are clear indications that many of those osberved in modern social environments prove harmful to individuals, and can be explained by compulsive tendencies. The innate desire for social validation that can be explained through evolutionary cues is far from what numerous individuals exhibit nowadays, especially since it is obviously paired with considerable detriment to their mental well-being. According to Volkow et al. (2009), addiction, in terms of neuroscience, is characterized by an imbalance in the dopaminergic system, with the consequence of altered dopamine release upon stimuli. While we will mainly assess substanceinduced changes in the neural wiring and functions, it will become increasingly obvious how many parallels we can draw. I will not even need to highlight them all, which I am sure of. Further, the increase in anticipatory drive (ibid.) is the source of the emergence of compulsive behavior. In an earlier study, Volkow et al. (2007) describe how drug-related stimuli reinforce cravings and the compulsive seeking for drugs, induced by elevated dopamine levels. Interestingly, Pascoli et al. (2018) show, how even in the face of adverse consequences (which are especially prominent and inevitable with prolonged substance abuse), the changes in synaptic plasticity in regions like the orbitofrontal cortex and the striatum solidify the persistence in drug-seeking. While that is, longterm substance abuse significantly diminishes the brain's responsiveness to the stimuli of rewards, a phenomenon known as *tolerance*, which causes an even more excessive focus on drug-related reinforcement, paired with a negligence of non-drug induced stimuli (Volkow et al., 2017). This is interesting in numerous regards: while the phenomenon of substance tolerance and diminishing responsiveness is widely known, we can bridge it seamlessly with the observations in societal dynamics: the growing need for validation and the ever-increasing sophistication in curated personas resemlbe the diminishing responsiveness to stimuli and the growing compulsion in perfection. Also, while the reinforcement of inferiority can shift the focus to the pursuit of perfection as an attempted counterbalance, paired with a shift to the personal insecurities and perceived inadequacies, it aligns perfectly with the dopamine-induced focus shift on drug (i.e. validation)-induced stimuli. I do not mean to say that this is the absolute same; I rather like to draw the attention to how well these phenomena integrate and work in unison. The increased focus on dopamine-hits finds its perfect basis in the focus shift on personal flaws, that is happening alongside. In a side-by-side comparison of drug-related compulsion and the compulsive pursuit of social validation, specifically in an attempt to mitigate the inner dissonance between the displayed perfection of peers and one's own shortcomings, there is little difference, after all.

The dysregulation in the dopamine system regularly leads to strong negative emotional states during withdrawal, fueling the behavior that strives to alleviate discomfort through dopamine pathways (Koob, 2008). Volkow et al.'s (2002) observations align with our previous establishments: even if the drug fails to provide pleasure (the *liking* aspect described by Schultz and Berridge & Robinson), the dopamine surge in the state of anticipation (the *wanting* aspect) leads to conditioning of cues and drive compulsive dopamine-seeking. Additionally, as we have mentioned, rational reasoning decreases under these compulsive drives, and it has been found, that this can probably be attributed to a decrease in function in the dopamine D2 receptor in the prefrontal cortex, which is the entity mainly involved in reasonable assessments (Volkow et al., 2009). Consequently, the brain's reward system is largely undermined, and rewired to compulsively seeking rewards, reinforcing drugrelated behaviors and prioritizing them over alternative ones (Dayan, 2009). In 2004, Koob et al. presented another interesting finding, where the 'brain plays another trick on us': through an additional engagement of the stress system, particularly the corticotropin-releasing factor (CRF), there is not only positive, but also negative reinforcement involved, which of course further strengthens the compulsion into the reward-seeking behavior spiral. As we have established earlier, negative reinforcement is another effective way of conditioning, where there is a negative consequence added upon undesired behavior instead of adding a positive one upon desired behavior. In combination, one can imagine the strength of such conditioning. Thus, the brain does not only phsically rewire toward reward-seeking behaviors, but does also 'punish' withdrawal through the release of stress transmitters, further entrenching the compulsion and forming a dysregulation spiral that is immensely hard to escape for the individual. As Gonzales & Weiss (1998) conclude, the perpetuation of maladaptive behaviors while at the same time reinforcing the ongoing dysregulation in the dopamine system makes it a complicated recovery process from addiction.

5.3 The Serotonergic System

5.3.1 Serotonin's Role and Mechanisms: A Brief Overview

This subchapter is meant to provide a concise overview of serotonin's general functions in the human brain, without yet linking it to the aforementioned dynamics. Firstly, serotonin is a key neurotransmitter involved in mood and emotional regulation and cognitive functions. Its regulation is critical for the maintenance of emotional stability, hence alterations in its levels can be directly linked to mental health disorders (Berger et al., 2009; Lucki, 1998). Its important role in several mood regulating and emotionally stabilizing processes in the brain was discovered mid 20th century. Kuhn (1958) highlighted serotonin's role especially through the discovery of tricyclic antidepressants, which was seminal for later research on its involvement in anxiety and depression. In 1967, Coppen published *The Biochemistry of Affective Disorders*, suggesting that a deficiency in serotonin levels contributes significantly to symptoms of depression, which became critical part of the foundational understanding of the biological rooting of depression. Moreover, the neurotransmitter is important for sleep cycles, appetite and even digestion. Disruptions in serotonin levels can cause insomnia and other significantly altered sleep-wake cycle patterns (Crockett et al., 2012), which is, apart from its direct influence on mood regulation, an important implication on secondary influence just as well. Long-term deprivation of sleep can heavily affect overall wellbeing. Serotonin's influence reaches into social behavior: Carver et al. (2008) were able to demonstrate that higher levels of serotonin can account for greater levels of empathy and promote social cooperation, while lower levels were associated with higher levels of aggression and impulsivity, thereby reducing social cognition and deteriorating social interactions in individuals. It plays a role in supporting neuroplasticity; low serotonin levels have been found to impair the brain's neuroplastic adaptive potential (Vaidya & Duman, 2001; Duman et al., 2016).

The majority of the brain's serotonin is produced in the raphe nuclei, located in the brain stem. From there, it is distributed across various brain regions, including amygdala, cortex and hippocampus. This widespread distribution explains its important roles in numerous critical brain and body functions (Müller & Jacobs, 2010). In the context of our examination, we will mainly focus on serotonin's role in mental well-being and especially shed light on its dynamics in interaction with dopamine, particularly in compulsive reward-seeking behaviors. However, to highlight its direct linking with mental health, it is valuable to evaluate key findings that contribute to our contemporary understanding of serotonin-linked mental disorders. In 2003, Caspi et al. found, that the gene 5-HTT, the 'Serotonin Transporter Gene', is an implicit indicator of genetic susceptibility to depression and related disorders. The regulation of anxiety is directly linked with serotonin levels, as has been established by Nutt et al. (2002), explaining that disorders like generalized anxiety disorder (GAD) and panic disorder can be caused by serotonin dysfunction. Likewise, serotonin influences repetitive and intrusive thoughts and behaviors in obsessive-compulsive disorder (OCD), which includes a wide range of symptoms, and hence makes serotonin-related medication (we will get into that soon) the first-line treatment for OCD. Furthermore, and especially interesting in light of our investigation, Angst (1986) could establish, that serotonin appears to play an important role in the mood cycling symptoms of bipolar disorder – *serotonin imbalances contribute significantly to the oscillation between manic and depressive states.*

Serotonin is predominantly synthesized in the brianstem's dorsal and median raphe (Lu et al., 2016). From there, serotonin neurons project throughout most of the brain, largely influencing areas like the hypothalamus, hippocampus, amygdala and the prefrontal cortex. In the cortex, serotonin is provided through the forebrain bundle, where it is responsible for influence on mood and cognition (Rubenstein, 1998), while through innervation of the hippocampus and modulation of large numbers of receptors, it regulates learning and memory (Berumen et al., 2012). In their 2022 work, Patodia et al. describe, how serotonin modulates motor control and reward processing in the basal ganglia, including the striatum and the substantia nigra. Further than that, it projects to the amygdala for the modulation of fear, anxiety and stress responses, in the hippocampal area it regulates emotionally charged situations. Through spinal pathways, it is also responsible for the perception of pain and further motor control (Pazos et al., 1987). Moreover, the so-called corticotropin-releasing hormones in the hypothalamus are influenced by serotonin from the raphe nuclei; thereby regulating the hypothalamic-pituitary-adrenal axis (HPA). Corticotropin release has been mentioned earlier, as an influential component in negative reinforcement processes during withdrawal from an addictive substance. Rubenstein (1998) has found, that serotonin is crucial for brain development, especially in terms of guiding neuronal differentiation and synapse formation during early neurogenesis. According to Sari (2004), who investigated the distribution of receptors 5-HT$_{1B}$ and 5-HT$_{2A}$, they are distributed widely across the cortex, hippocampus and basal ganglia. Nugent et al. (2013) further mention the 5-HT$_{1A}$ receptor interacting with serotonin in order to reduce anxiety and stabilize mood in its action in the hippocampus and the cortex.

Our main focus for the transition into dopamine-serotonin balances is the important influence in mood regulation that serotonin exhibits, especially through analysis of the effects in dysregulation and integration of the knowledge in neuropsychopharmacology. Because chemical treatment of serotonin levels is directly linked with the knowledge about its initial distribution and the large influence it exercises on several key functions in the brain, we will examine those parts as one whole perspective. The three main parts I would like to highlight are the following:

1. *Mood Stabilization Process via Serotonin*
2. *Serotonin's Role in Stress Management*
3. *Serotonin's Role in Processing Emotional Stimuli.*

As already mentioned, through interaction with the so-called 5-HT receptors distributed throughout the brain, serotonin is critical for regulating mood and providing emotional stability. When serotonin binds to 5-HT_{1A} receptors, it activates signaling cascades, that inhibit excessive release of excitatory neurotransmitters, like glutamate. Did that not happen, the uncontrolled release of such would end in excessive stress, anxiety and panic due to the overactivity in stress- and emotion related neural circuits. This mechanism allows for a balanced mood state (Celada et al., 2013). On the other hand, serotoninergic modulation of neuroplasticity is an important action for maintaining the emotional flexibility to react on different situations, most of all through promotion of the growth of new neurons in the hippocampus (i.e. *neurogenesis*), which strengthens those synaptic connections that are essential for emotional resilience and reduces the vulnerability for mood disorders (Duman & Aghajanian, 2012; Jenkins et al., 2016).

Secondly, as mentioned, serotonin possesses the ability to regulate the brain's response to stressors. Through influencing the HPA, which governs stress responses, it helps inhibiting excessive cortisol production in the body. Whenever the brain receives a stressing stimulus, the amygdala signals the hypothalamus to activate the HPA axis, which results in the release of cortisol. Through intercation with the 5-HT_{1A} receptors, serotonin serves as a 'buffer' preventing the brain from uncontrolled release of cortisol (Harmer, 2008; Mandelli et al., 2007).

Lastly, serotonin's effect on specific emotional circuits that influence how we perceive and interpret emotional information, accounts for its importance in regulating our subsequent reactions to emotional stimuli. When serotonin binds to 5-HT_{2A} receptors in the amygdala, it can attenuate its reaction to emotional stimuli, specifically necessary for the processing of fear and emotional salience. The result of binding to these receptors is avoidance of hypervigilance and overreaction, specifically to stimuli that would otherwise be perceived as threatening (Gillihan et al., 2010; Mehrens et al., 2007). In the prefrontal cortex, serotonin helps exerting top-down control over the amygdala through the integration of higher-order thinking in the assessment of emotional stimuli, balancing emotional responses and ensuring tempered and appropriate reactions through reason. This is also an important factor in the prevention of mood swings and emotional dysregulation (Ressler & Nemeroff, 2000). Furthermore, according to Harmer et al. (2006), balanced serotonin can reduce the attention bias toward negative information, which is an important state of focus to prevent the onset of anxiety or depression disorders.

Serotonin has a major function in the regulation of sleep and wake cycles, which is indirectly partially responsible for a well-balanced mood *through sleep*. According to Snyder et al. (2006), signals from the suprachiasmatic nucleus, which can be described as the brains 'biological clock', are responsible for a chemical process that converts serotonin to melatonin, a derivative of it, that influences metabolic rhythms. Through modulation of the oscillatory levels of 5-HT *N-acetyltransferase* melatonin production and amplitudes are controlled in order to respond to environmental signals of day and night (ibid.). Serotonin is thus first acetylated to form N acetylserotonin, then methylated by *hydroxyindole-O-methyltransferase* to produce melatonin. The environmental light is an important factor, since it has been established, that especially blue light is an inhibitor of melatonin production (Szewczyk et al., 2018). Low light conditions however foster the production of melatonin – the rising levels of serotonin during the day can be seen as preparation to synthesis into melatonin for the night, ensuring that the circadian rhythm remains somewhat synchronized with environmental light and dark cycles (Takahashi, 1991). The important function of serotonin for the later synthesis into melatonin is a crucial aspect, since low levels of serotonin can be directly responsible for problematically low melatonin production and subsequently sleep disturbances, especially a prolonged onset latency (Leu-Semenescu et al., 2010; Roseboom et al., 1996; Maurizi, 1990). Moreover, it has been found that serotonin availability does not only significantly influence melatonin synthesis but also the sleep-wake cycle itself (Vollrath et al., 1988).

5.3.2 Pathology of Serotonin Depletion With Insights From Neuropsychopharmacology: Selective Serotonin Reuptake Inhibitors

Low serotonin levels are strongly linked to the development of major depressive disorder. Insufficiency in serotonin does not only lead to the brain's failure to regulate mood and thereby persistent feelings of hopelessness, sadness and loss of interest (Cowen, 1993; Coppen & Doogan, 1988), but also shift the brain's bias toward negativity and impair its counterbalancing function so the focus is strongly on negative stimuli, being linked to aggression and even suicidal tendencies (Coccaro, 1989; Narvaes et al. 2014; Sadkowski et al., 2013). As a major source of self-sustenance in depression, receptor sensitivity changes and serotonin transporters are less active in the brain, both of which contribute to the prolonging and exacerbation of symptoms; leading to reduced avaliability of serotonin in critical brain regions and also weakening the brain's response to it (Bligh-Glover et al., 2000; Meltzer, 1990). Typically, cognitive functions are affected through diminishing synaptic plasticity, for which serotonin is crucial. This eventually results in impaired memory and decision making (Jenkins et al., 2016). Since serotonin is primarily a stabilizing element, inhibiting strong emotional outbursts (Carver et al., 2008), it consequently leads to poor control over one's emotions when serotonin levels are low. Irritability is increased, leading to impulsivity, hostility and inability to proper reaction on stimuli (Coccaro, 1989).

From a psychological perspective, major depressive disor-

der (MDD), commonly referred to as depression, is characterized by a range of symptoms, whereas it should be distinguished from just colloquial terms of natural mood alterations
in response to life's circumstances. The American Psychological Association (APA), in their diagnostic manual, characterizes MDD as a persistent low mood and sadness for a minimum of two weeks (APA, 2013). One of the key features of
pathological depression is the diminished capacity to excperience pleasure, especially through those that had previously
brought joy. This is called *anhedonia* (King, 2002). It is a
common symptom, that individuals suffering from depression
think particularly poorly of themselves, often accompanied by
feelings of guilt or self-responsibility for the array of negative
feelings (Beck, 1976); those are common cognitive distortions,
that are part of the so-called cognitive triad: poor opinions
of oneself, of one's surroundings (including other individuals)
and the own future, or the future in general. Those feelings
often tie together and are inseparable from one another, so
that the individual may feel an overwhelming sense of sadness,
guilt, worthlessness, hopelessness with a general tendency to
attribute undue blame for it all to themselves (APA, 2013).

MDD can disrupt sleep patterns and result in both insomnia or, its opposite, hypersomnia (Nutt et al., 2008). This is a
particularly vicious cycle, as sleep is essential for mental well-
being in the first place. As MDD disrupts circadian rhythms
and can cause heavily detrimental effects on sleep patterns,
it is another means of self-sustenance since poor sleep further
fuels and exacerbates the mood. Results are often characteristic for MDD: a general feeling of fatigue with considerable
decrease in overall energy levels, which hinders the individual in engagement in daily activities, impacting one's sense
of accomplishment and also causing social withdrawal (APA,
2013). Especially, the sense of general fatigue is an important
implicator of psychomotor changes, including either agitation
or retardation (Parker, 2005). This can be one of the reasons, why even simple tasks feel particularly physically taxing, causing further refrain from activity. According to King

(2002), it is due to the pervasive sense of hopelessness, that individuals often tend to become suicidal or at least develop suicidal thoughts. Joiner et al. (2006) see social withdrawal as a consequence of the abundance of symptoms, and likewise as a significant contributor to their exacerbation. An amplified sense of isolation is understandably a foundation for further drift from reality in a sense of distortion that tells an individual 'all is lost'.

It is not uncommon for depression to co-occur with obsessive-compulsive disorder (OCD), particularly in the context of serotonin dysregulation, where symptoms of both conditions may overlap and exacerbate one another. Comorbidity of depression is believed to make 39.5% in OCD patients (Tükel et al., 2002). OCD is characterized by persistent and intrusive thoughts or urges (obsessions) that can lead to significant emotional distress (APA, 2013). Given the varying severity and wide range of symptoms associated with OCD, I will focus on the compulsive thoughts and associated patterns, as this aligns more closely with our current context and connects seamlessly with the broader concepts of this work. While in OCD, the compulsive thoughts and obsessions are unwanted and often irrational, individuals often feel powerless to control or even disregard them (Clark, 2004). In comorbidity with major depressive disorder, the latter has been found to exacerbate compulsive symptoms, which leads to increased functional impairment (Viswanath et al., 2012). Individuals may compulsively end up in spiralling thoughts and compulisve cycles of overthinking, while the topics often center around fears related to some kind of harm or moral violations and similar topics, contributing to increased anxiety (Rachman, 1997). Moreover, in the combination with the high likelihood to develop overlapping symptoms with other low-serotonin associated states, patients often find themselves in cycles of obsessive spiralling that intensify the suffering and depressive ruminations, leading to perpetuation of the focus and bias in negativity. According to the APA (2013), such individuals often choose to engage in repetitive behavioral patterns or mental processes to cope with the distressing compulsions and which are intended to alleviate the perceived anxiety. It is not rare, that the exhibited patterns provide some sort of relief experience, but subsequently exacerbate the compulsion itself, in a pattern of self-sustenance; consequently, the disorder becomes particularly difficult to overcome and the thinking patterns become increasingly obsessive, ever gravitating back to the compulsion (Abramowitz, 2006; Salkovskis, 1985). Specifically, impairment of concentration is a common consequence of the high cognitive load that patients develop. As a result, treatment becomes more challenging, because the cycle is continuously reinforced (Perugi et al., 1997). As in depression, cognitive distortions play a major role in OCD. As we have established, serotonin's role transcends beyond stabilization of mood and is involved in critical processes in the brain in the evaluation of fear and anxiety and helps regulate reactions to perceived threats. Thus, individuals with manifested OCD often exhibit behavioral patterns that (to them) ensure, that mistakes or transgressions have not occured (Abramowitz et al., 2006); maintain perfectionistic standards, thereby exacerbating their own obsessive overthinking (Frost & Steketee, 2002). According to Rachman (2002) it is a common symptom that OCD patients have a heightened sense of responsibility, growing in the belief that through their compulsion, it is their obligation to prevent negative outcomes. This, on the other hand, further heightens ther innate anxiety, because it becomes a self-fueling cycle of maladaptation, where the patients attempt to exert utmost control in an effort to manage perceived threats (Purdon & Clark, 2002). Lastly, anxiety is believed to be the main connector between both conditions (Perugi et al., 1997). Typically, the treatment involves so-called selective serotonin reuptake inhibitors (SSRI), alongside cognitive-behavioral therapy (Brady, 2014). At this point, we will see how crucial the prior elaborations in neurochemical interconnections were, since it is a clear path we are following in understanding the intricate relationships between societal circumstances and dynamics, behavioral science, neurobiology, psychology and the essential neurochemical foundations for our psychological perspectives.

Selective serotonin reuptake inhibitors primarily function by inhibiting the serotonin transporter (SERT), which is a protein located in the presynaptic membrane and plays a critical role in the reabsorption of serotonin. This reabsorption happens from the synaptic cleft back into the presynaptic neuron for future release (Hirano et al., 2005). SSRI bind to SERT proteins and effectively prevent the reabsorption, which increases serotonin availability in the synaptic space (Xue et al., 2016). *Selective* in SSRI refers to their strong affinity to target serotonin over other neurotransmitters like dopamine or norepinephrine, making them particularly effective in the treatment for mood regulation (Sokolowski & Seiden, 1999). The particular effectiveness is grounded in the fact, that under normal circumstances, serotonin is rapidly cleared from the synapse by the transporting protein SERT; thus, the increase in extracellular serotonin enhances the chance of it binding to postsynaptic receptors – prolonged presence of serotonin in the synaptic space facilitates higher amounts and sustenance of signaling instead of absorption (Kulikov et al., 2018; Kim et al., 2002). While that is, the latter have also found that higher serotonin levels trigger syntheses of *tryptophan hydroxylase*, which enhances serotonergic signaling. Generally, with more available serotonin that is not reabsorbed, *postsynaptic 5-HT receptors* are obviously more frequently activated. Their specific modulation functions have been elaborated previously; most importantly, 5-HT_{1A} and 5-HT_{2A} receptors are targeted, while activation of the 5-HT_{1A} is particularly associated with anxiolytic and antidepressant effects. This in turn helps modulate stress responses more effectively, reducing overreactions and regulating the release of stress hormones like cortisol. With this mechanism, all regulation processes in the different brain regions affected through serotonin depletion, can unfold; anxiety is reduced, stress levels decrease, cognitive reasoning is enhanced. Lastly, long-term SSRI treatment has been associated with the promotion of neuroplasticity, exhibiting enduring changes in synaptic structures. This happens through stimulation of *brain-derived neurotrophic factor (BDNF)*, a protein that is crucial for neuron survival and also formation of new synapses. SSRIs have been found to especially promote that process in the hippocampus (Kulikov et al., 2018). Moreover, BDNF is important in the reversal of synaptic atrophy happening as an effect of MDD, where chronically high stress levels diminish the number of synaptic connections (Oh et al., 2018); this could be understood as the opposite of neuroplasticity (Duman & Duman, 2015; Qiao et al., 2017; Licinio & Wong, 2002). These proven effects in SSRIs associate them with greater cognitive flexibility and better emotional responses after onset of their enhancement in neuroplasticity. Since we know, how structural enhancements of the brains circuits can not only foster learning and cognitive adaptation, but are also a critical part of emotional regulation, it is understood, that they do contribute to balancing effects in mood through plasticity-enhancements.

5.3.3 Serotonin's Functions in Social Environments

Serotonin is integral to the regulation of social behavior and the perception of hierarchy, acting as a mediator of social status and also modulating emotional responses to social cues. Research indicates that serotonin is accountible for the modulation of behavior that is associated with balancing dominance versus submission. While higher levels of serotonin are associated with increased affiliative behaviors and reduced levels of aggression, low serotonin levels diminish social cognition and can be a source of social aggression (Edwards & Kravitz, 1997). Evidenced across various species, individuals with lower concentration of 5-HIAA (a metabolite of serotonin) in their cerebrospinal fluid, tend to display higher levels of aggression (Linnoila & Virkkunen, 1992). However, there is an aspect that needs clarification. Firstly, the fact that serotonin has strong implications for perception of social status and dynamics in social heirarchies is an essential observation, since it ties in our previously elaborated concept of inferiority and coping mechanisms. Secondly, the relationship between serotonin, aggression and social dominance is complex. As mentioned, low levels of serotonin can be affiliated with aggression, however, although counterintuitive, those individuals displaying dominance in social environments are those with *higher* serotonin levels. It is important not to confuse *dominance* and *aggression*; the display of dominance correlates with higher serotonin levels for several reasons. Individuals with higher levels of serotonin tend to be more self-confident and less doubtful about themselves, have a greater emotional balance and display assertiveness without resorting to aggression. The emotional balance and the higher level of social cognition mentioned before are reasons, that they have reduced levels of anxiety and less potential to overreact to perceived threats (Carver et al., 2008; Tse & Bond, 2002; Higley et al., 1996). While in the emotional framework of individuals with low serotonin levels, there may be higher needs for a compensatory response to hierarchical order and social subordination, it is the higher level of serotonin that encourages self-confidence and assertiveness without the need for aggressive enforcement. Furthermore, certain genetic variants of the serotonin transporter gene 5-HTT have been linked to higher responsiveness to social status cues and better adaptation to hierarchical structures (Canli & Lesch, 2007). These adaptations and social integration without aggressive potential, obviously, lead to better social harmony and group cohesion, supporting one's social interactions. From that perspective, it works bidirectional, because research indicates that positive social interactions in turn foster serotonin signaling in the brain (Kiser et al., 2012) – reinforcing affiliative behavior and thus more positive signaling. On the other hand, exhibiting antisocial behavioral patterns paired with social aggression leads to the opposite and can certainly create a negative cycle of reinforcement with negative social cues.

5.4 The Complex Antagonistic Relationship Between Serotonin and Dopamine

5.4.1 Dopamine and Serotonin Receptor Interaction: Competitive Reciprocal Inhibition

With dopamine receptors (D1-D5) mainly distributed in the striatum, nucleus accumbens prefrontal cortex and the ventral tegmental area, and serotonin receptors mainly distributed in the raphe nuclei, hippocampus, but also in the prefrontal cortex and ventral tegmental area (Alex & Pehek, 2007; Bubar et al., 2007), and their roles that are distinct from each other, there are still numerous interactions between the two neurotransmitters that are noteworthy in our context. As they function in reciprocal modulation and even in an inhibitory manner, we will explore, how dopamine-seeking behavior can eventually cause serotonin depletion, leading to an array of symptoms that we clarified in the last chapter.

The activation of serotonin 5-HT$_{2C}$ receptors in the VTA modulates dopamine neurotransmission through inhibition of GABAergic interneurons. Activity of those dopamine neurons is tightly regulated by GABAergic interneurons exerting inhibitory control over them (Huidobro-Toro et al., 1996). Thus, when 5-HT$_{2C}$ receptors are activated, they 'disinhibit' dopamine release, through inhibiting GABA interneurons capable of restricting dopamine neurons (Alex & Pehek, 2007; Valencia-Torres et al., 2017). This however is a highly nuanced process, since modulation of the VTA's output can be graded just to the needed level of GABAergic inhibition, hardening or softening dopamine neurotransmission (Liu et al., 2003).

Without going into utmost and painstaking detail in the large number of findings that have limited relevance for our own argumentation, I would rather like to cite a notable study conducted by Niederkofler et al. (2015), presenting highly sophisticated details on the mutual innervations and distributions of dopaminergic and serotonergic neurons across the brain. In their study *Functional Interplay Between Dopaminergic and Serotonergic Neuronal Systems During Development and Adulthood*, they explain:

> Until recently, most research has been aimed at understanding the function of these neurotransmitter systems independently. However, a growing body of evidence supports the notion that to fully comprehend the brain, we must understand the way that various neural systems interact. [...] Both mDA and 5-HT neurons receive input from neural regions distributed throughout the brain, conveying information about a veriety of different functional processes. Notably, tracing and immunohistochemical studies demonstrate that many of the afferent inputs into select mDA and 5-HT nuclei originate from the same neural regions [...] highlighting the potential coregulation of both neurotransmitter systems and accounting for the considerable overlap in affective and cognitive functions influenced by each system. [...] The anatomical proximity and common projection targets of the mDA and 5-HT neurotransmitter systems in the adult brain positions them to impact similar physiological and behavioral processes. Indeed, the two systems are known to modulate many of the same, yet very diverse, behaviors and processes, such as aggression, reward processing, and locomotion. As we shall see, it is becoming increasingly apparent that the comodulation of these processes involves, to some extens, an interaction between mDA and 5-HT neurons. (Niederkofler et al., 2015).

In light of these elaborations, I will present an array of supporting arguments, that solidify the idea, that the unprecedented extent in validation seeking which modern individuals exhibit and that are amplified by the equally unprecedented digital environments and trends we learned earlier, have strong implications for the brain's dopamine-, and thereby, serotonin dynamics.

5.4.2 Dopamine Spike-Induced Serotonin-Depleting Feedback Loops

Dopamine spikes trigger a series of feedback mechanisms that influence both dopamine and serotonin signaling. When dopamine levels surge, feedback inhibition pathways are activated, which means that dopamine receptors adjust their sensitivity through phosphorylation mechanisms – a process that modifies proteins in the cell to regulate their function. Phosphorylation of dopamine receptors, especially D2 receptors, leads to an adaptive response where receptor sensitivity is modulated to avoid overactivation. This, in turn, modulates synaptic activity, affecting how neurons communicate with each other (Nishi et al., 2000). A key aspect of this process is the activation of dopamine D2 receptors, which are a specific type of dopamine receptor that plays a direct role in reducing serotonin signaling by inhibiting the excitability of serotonin neurons, effectively making them less likely to fire (Aman et al., 2007). In regions like the dorsal raphe nucleus, D2 receptor activation inhibits serotonin neuron activity indirectly, reducing serotonergic output. This interaction again highlights the antagonistic relationship between dopamine and serotonin, where increased dopamine disrupts serotonergic transmission, particularly in key brain regions associated with emotional regulation and mood stabilization (Winterer et al., 2011).

Further, dopamine spikes initiate downregulation of serotonin receptor activity via protein kinase pathways – another cellular mechanism that reduces the ability of serotonin to signal between neurons – contributing to a reduction in serotonin transmission (Parga et al., 2007). In particular, Protein Kinase C (PKC) and Protein Kinase A (PKA) are involved in phsphorylating serotonin receptors, leading to receptor desensitization and reduced serotonin transmission. This feedback mechanism is especially prevalent in the nucleus accumbens, where the interaction of dopamine D1 and D2 receptors modulates serotonin release, amplifying the effect of dopamine on serotonin signaling (Rahman & McBride, 2001). Additionally, the modulation of glutamatergic activity by dopamine D1 receptors in the NAc plays a role in enhancing dopamine-driven neurotransmission, further reducing serotonin's influence in reward processing. Serotonin 5-HT_{2C} receptors, which normally inhibit dopamine release as a regulatory mechanism, are influenced by elevated dopamine, further weakening serotonin's ability to regulate dopamine levels (De Deurwaerdère et al., 2004). Clarification: remembering from the previous section, where 5-HT_{2C} receptors were specifically mentioned in the context of disinhibiting dopamine release, this is not a contradiction: in most brain regions (particularly the striatum and NAc), 5-HT_{2C} do indeed inhibit dopamine release, however in the VTA, the process is somewhat inversed through the involvement of GABAergic interneurons; since they restrict dopamine activity.

Through these phosphorylation dynamics, dopamine spikes diminish serotonin-mediated signaling, with long-loop feedback circuits extending their influence to mesocortical systems – meaning that these effects are not just localized but spread to higher-order brain regions involved in complex functions like cognition and decision-making (Schultz, 2002; Pehek & Hernan, 2015). The mesocortical pathway, which connects the VTA to the PFD, is crucial in regulating executive functions like decision-making and impulse control. Prolonged dopamine elevation in this pathway suppresses serotonin's stabilizing effect on cognition, making higher-order functions more dopamine-driven overall. Dopamine also interacts with glutamatergic pathways at synaptic junctions (the main communication areas of neurons), reducing serotonin efficacy when dopamine is elevated (Zhong et al., 2008). This cross-talk between the two neurotransmitters contributes to an overall suppression of serotonin transmission, especially when dopamine activity is heightened, further affecting mood and behavior. This reduction in serotonin's ability to modulate glutamatergic synapses affects synaptic plasticity, leading to reduced flexibility in emotional and cognitive processes.

During periods characterized by heightened reward-seeking behavior, increased dopamine levels can inhibit serotonin transmission through the modulation of synaptic plasticity, particularly within the NAc, a critical area for reward processing (Fiorino et al., 1993). This indicates that the brain's capacity to adapt and reinforce specific neural connections in response to rewards is influenced, with dopamine taking precedence over serotonin. Dopamine's dominance in modulating plasticity in the NAc shifts reward learning processes toward dopaminergic control, reducing serotonin's contribution to reward evaluation. Elevated dopamine levels activate D2 receptors, which directly dampen the excitability of serotonin neurons, consequently reducing the likelihood of serotonin release (Aman et al., 2007). This interaction leads to a decrease in serotonin availability, thereby lessening its impact on mood regulation.

As Niederkofler stated, dopamine and serotonin utilize overlapping neural pathways and engage in competitive signaling. A surge in dopamine levels diminishes serotonin's effectiveness (Nakazato, 2019), which is particularly observed in the striatum, where elevated dopamine inhibits serotonin's ability to influence reward-related behavior (Yoshimoto et al., 1999). This competitive signaling is particularly strong in dopaminergic-driven circuits, where serotonin's inhibitory role over impulsivity is weakened. In the mesolimbic system – an integral to reinforcement and reward – high dopamine levels not only amplify dopamine-mediated reinforcement but also actively suppress serotonergic modulation, resulting in an imbalance in reward and mood regulation (Rocha et al., 2002). In addition, it has been found that the frequent spikes in dopamine activate cross-inhibitory feedback loops in brain regions such as the NAc and dorsal raphe, further diminishing serotonin release (Fudge & Emiliano, 2003). These feedback circuits shift the balance towards dopaminergic dominance, particularly in the PFC, crucial for decision-making and impulse control (Ferenczi et al., 2016). Dopamine's influence in the PFC alters the balance between impulsivity and regulation, as serotonin's modulating effects are increasingly suppressed during repeated reward-seeking behaviors and episodes. As dopamine predominates in these pathways, serotonin receptor sensitivity declines further, rendering serotonin less effective (McBride et al., 1990). In summary, prolonged elevation of dopamine results in sustained inhibitory effects on serotonin circuits, which means that even after dopamine levels normalize, serotonin's capacity to influence mood and behavior remains impaired (Miyazaki et al., 2014). Especially the desensitization of 5-HT_{1A} and 5-HT_{2A} receptors leads to diminished mood-regulating efficacy, making individuals more prone to impulsive and reward-driven behaviors. This long-term suppression can lead to increased impulsivity and even more pronounced reward-seeking behaviors, as serotonin's role in inhibiting such actions is sustainably diminished (Soubrié, 1986).

A notable 2011 study by Boureau and Dayan, called *Opponency Revisited: Competition and Cooperation Between Dopamine and Serotonin*, shows, that the competitive inhibition of dopamine and serotonin is highly complex, with observations being highly dependent on the brain region. They specifically refer to studies by Berridge (2007) and Gruninger et al. (2007) in their explanation of dopamine and serotonin standing in a competitive relationship in 'appetite vs. satiation', meaning engaging in behavior vs. ending behavior in this context. However, they also state the complexity of action-reaction patterns not only across neurons and neurotransmitters, but even single receptor types:

> Indeed, 5-HT_{2C} receptors in general tonically inhibit DA release. However, many 5-HT receptor types (5-HT_{1A}, 5-HT_{2A}, 5-HT_{3A}, 5-HT_{4A}) stimulate DA release (Alex and Peehek, 2007; Di Matteo et al, 2008; Higgins and Fletcher, 2003), and

5-HT generally seems to exert an excitatory influence on the VTA (Beart and McDonald, 1982;
Van Bockstaele et al, 1994), including enhancing
DA release in the nucleus accumbens (Guan and
McBride, 1989). The opposition between 5-HT$_{2A}$
and 5-HT$_{2C}$ seems particularly striking. Both receptor types have been shown to display constitutive activity (Berg et al, 2005; De Deurwaerdère
et al, 2004; Navailles et al, 2006), and exert opposite control over the release of DA in the nucleus accumbens and striatum (Porras et al, 2002;
Di Giovanni et al, 1999; De Deurwaerdère and
Spampinato, 1999) and in the PFC (Millan et al,
1998; Gobert et al, 2000; Pozzi et al, 2002; Alex
et al, 2005; Pehek et al, 2006). 5-HT has a critical role in modulating impulsivity, perhaps partly
indirectly by modulating DA release (Dalley et
al, 2002, 2008; Winstanley et al, 2004, 2006; Millan et al, 2000a). Indeed, these effects may result in the behavioral observation that 5-HT$_{2A}$ receptors are associated with increased impulsivity,
whereas 5-HT$_{2C}$ activity displays the more general correlation of 5-HT with decreased impulsivity (Robinson et al, 2008; Winstanley et al, 2004;
Fletcher et al, 2007). Effects of 5-HT$_{2C}$ appear to
be mediated by receptors at the level of the origin (VTA) for PFC DA (Alex et al, 2005; Pozzi
et al, 2002), the target (striatum) for dorsolateral
striatal DA (Alex et al, 2005), and both for the nucleus accumbens (Navailles et al, 2008). (Boureau
& Dayan, 2001, p. 83).

In conclusion, it becomes clear, how delicate the relationship between dopamine and serotonin is in the brain, and
also, that there is much more to be explored in the explicit
dynamics they exhibit in their cross-communication. It is
not only the neurotransmitters alone, but also the competition and overlap in pathways, and sometimes the counterin-

tuitive effect that activation of either receptors can have, that make the bidirectional effects highly complex in nature. However, despite the complexity, we can now confidently propose, that overly frequent and significant dopamine surges lead to a strain on serotonin and its receptor functions, thereby drastically reducing serotonin's ability to regulate mood and stabilize emotional responses. The self-sustaining cycle that erupts in the brain leads to further uncontrolled and compulsive dopamine-seeking, because the inhibitory control instance diminishes further. This paves the way for serious mental challenges, and the overarching notion becomes clear: constant dopamine overload undermines serotonin's counterbalance and disrupts emotional stability.

6 INTEGRATING NEUROCHEMICAL DYSREGULATION IN MODERN VALIDATION-SEEKING

Dopamine-mediated reward systems in the brain that originally served to secure social bonds for survival have long expanded to seeking external approval in far broader social circles and way beyond local peer groups; they operate on the neural principles humans have inherited from ancestry, but they do no longer serve the same purposes. Rather, they have come to serve their own mechanisms nowadays, sustaining the pursuit of ever more validation.

Sherman et al. (2016; 2018) conducted fMRI imaging and were able to find, that social media validation, such as receipt of likes, stimulates the same brain regions as other reward processing, including the striatum and the NAc. Dopamine release could thus be linked to validation received from social media, resembling the reward obtained. Through this positive feedback signaling, the online behavior is reinforced and encourages repetitive engagement with the platform the validation originated from. Moreover, the anticipatory dopamine release during social media interactions reflects the patterns described in variable reinforcement schedules, since the unpredictability therein reinforces reward-seeking behaviors (Meshi et al., 2013; Fiorillo et al., 2003; Rosenthal-von der Pütten et al., 2019).

In 2021, Marengo et al. confirmed, that likes on social media act as variable reinforcement, where unpredictable feedback triggers dopamine release, encouraging users to seek the same rewards more consistently. Interestingly, the behavior that can be observed in social networks is tied closely to the social learning behavior explained earlier, with those individuals more sensitive to social feedback showing greater potential to alter their behavior online, based on the estimation of further likes (Fareri & Delgado, 2014). The methodical exploitation of these mechanisms, which is not a main part of this work, still significantly exacerbates this behavior, in favor of the platforms and their monetary interests; while we have a different focus in this argumentation, it still underlines the efficacy with which the dopamine circuitry can be addressed through the distribution of virtual social validation (Wadsley et al., 2021; Gross et al., 2024).

I would like to explain, that the reasons here tie together seamlessly. While there are indeed strong financial incentives to keep users engaged on a platform, and on the other hand, we know that the tech companies maintaining these platforms are in fact among the wealthiest companies in the world and in the entire history of humanity, the precision and effectiveness with which they tap into human neuropsychological frameworks is stunning. Mobile services and apps receive frequent updates 'enhancing the user experience'. Nowadays, entire industries are centered around enhancements of interfaces in mobile devices and apps, which has to monetize in some way. It would not make sense to launch an app with an incredibly expensive background in development, testing, and an ever-so sophisticated user experience, if using the app were for free, without subscription or any other means of compensation for the company behind it. Thus, the constant enhancements and the amount of research dedicated to 'user experience' is nothing else than creating the most intuitive and captivizingly-engaging way to spend time on the platform and engulf in the experiences triggering the mechanism that maintains one's constant engagement. Monetized through highly targeted advertising, selected and curated by algorithms several times more capable than the most precise humanly made personality analyses, individuals are targeted by advertising content in real-time, all the time. The net worth of the major social media companies speaks for itself, hence we do not need any more confirmation that the model works and pays off. What does that mean for human behavior?

The bidirectional and non-arbitrary way this works means that devices, platforms and virtually the entire environment around those social networks is highly intuitive and tailored to encourage users to continue with their behavior in seeking validation (i.e. rewards), which of course solidifies the patterns, since all the features are targeted to tap into this exact behavior. Little does is surprise in light of these sophistications, that users appear to fully intuitively immerse themselves in these networks, compulsively glued to their screens. In this regard, it is obvious how on the one hand, users actively seek to activate their devices, in order to be provided with a dopamine hit, and on the other hand they *are sought* to, by careful design. In everyday life, social networks provide users with quick, frequent dopamine spikes through various forms of validation, such as likes, comments, and notifications. Every time a user receives a like or a new follower, the brain's reward system is activated, specifically the dopamine pathways in the ventral striatum and nucleus accumbens. These dopamine surges occur not just when the reward is received but also in anticipation of it. For example, when users post a picture or status update, they are already anticipating the feedback, which triggers dopamine even before the actual likes come in.

The unpredictability of when and how much social feedback will be received – resembling a variable reward schedule – further strengthens the reward-seeking behavior. Users check their phones frequently, in anticipation of that next burst of validation, driven by the possibility of unexpected notifications. This pattern is reinforced over time as the brain links the behavior of engaging with the platform to the dopamine release, creating a habit loop. Here, the design is at play:

through utmost planning in each slight detail of the app, creators ensure that each action, even the motion of skimming through the platform's contents, is intuitive and supports the solidifying habit. The frequent checking of one's smartphone is not even a fully conscious action anymore, and often has no specific purpose but is rather a reinforced motion, that appears to melt with other fully natural behavioral patterns. In a 2020 study of 526 participants, Beierle et al. found, that on average, users would check their smartphones 72 times per day. While many of those checks have no specific purpose, it can also be mere environmental triggers rather than fully deliberate actions that account for the checks (Oulasvirta et al., 2012), and would often be prompted by even the shortest streaks of boredom throughout daily routines (Elhai et al., 2017). There is an element that can remind one of smoking cigarettes, here not in the sense of substance addiction that is, but in the combination of the psychological element of bridging a short while with the habitual motion of the hands, keeping mind and body a little busy. It is commonly known that many cigarette smokers have reported, while attempting to quit, that the actual habit of holding the cigarette in their fingers is a substantial part of the addiction. Oulasvirta et al. (2012) have adopted the unaware and automatic nature of taking up the phone and checking it frequently is a habitual behavior very similar to addiction pathways. This can culminate in attention 'hijacking', where users pick up the phones and check their platforms for new notifications unconsciously, even during critical tasks like driving (Farmer et al., 2015). This aligns with the findings from a study published by Billieux et al. (2015), who argue, that the characteristics of these actions strongly remind of compulsive disorders, where the urge to perform the action actually overrides the awareness of the action itself. In 2016, Zheng & Lee stated, that even the silent and in-background notifications trigger the urges to check for new stimulations, triggering the unpredictable reinforcement in dopamine-driven feedback loops through creating a perpetual state of '*there could be a new re-*

ward for me'. These actions however, are not fully conscious and over time, solidify themselves as automatic and unaware routines replicating multiple times throughout the day. Tying back to the reward circuitry in the brain, individuals learn that this is behavior possibly linked to reward, so they should keep engaged.

What we see is a nature of frequent spikes in dopamine, introduced by intermittent social validation in digital form, but it reveals its detrimental nature only after a while. There is solid scientific evidence for a *spike-crash* nature in dopamine surges, that we are elborating on here. This means, that the frequent surges in dopamine are motivational boosters, providing feelings of joy and pleasure, but this has a rebound effect. Not only is it the tolerance I mentioned, which is a state of receptor desensitization over time, resulting in a so-called *hypodopaminergic state*, where the reinforcers that priorly excited the release of large amounts of dopamine are no longer satisfying (Volkow et al., 2002). It is the oscillating nature of chronic spikes in dopamine that brings about a rebound effect where elevated dopamine levels crash and induce a strong sense of dissatisfaction that is followed by a craving for the next dopamine hit (Lembke, as cited in Hu & Nguyen, 2022). This permanent oscillation is the reason why anything in overindulgence can potentially become addictive. Dopamine release is not substance-bound, as to think the human brain might regulate these oscillations itself. While there is, indeed, the mechanism of serotonin counteracting the overload in dopamine *at first*, as we have established, it is only a matter of time until this control instance becomes obsolete and ineffective. As dopamine takes increasing precedence over serotonin as its antagonist, there is little impulse control, giving way to the next reward-driven cycle. As brain structures adapt to the frequent release of *phasic* dopamine – the sort released in response or elevated anticipatory excitement to reward, other than *tonic* dopamine, available in lower concentrations as the baseline in the synaptic cleft (Grace, 2000) – serotonin depletes and loses its control activity. Rastogi et al. (1977) found this effect in the context of withdrawal from benzodiazepine treatment, and could attribute the rebound to dopamine dynamics, solidifying these findings.

The described rebound can be attributed to the amplitudinal surges and dips of dopamine in response to rewarding stimuli or their anticipation: after the surge in dopamine wears off, the levels dip below the baseline, which is often referred to as *crash*. The period of the crash, which is defined by dopamine levels below the baseline, that have to only gradually reestablish again, is characterized for the individual by low motivation levels, reduced pleasure up to anhedonia and a sense of dissatisfaction (Kringelbach & Berridge, 2010; Koob & Le Moal, 2001; Volkow et al., 2010). The aforementioned desensitization, in combination with other neuroadaptive changes in the brain's wiring, contributes to withdrawal-like symptoms during the rebound, known from substance addiction (Koob & Le Moal, 1997). Known as *hedonic dysregulation*, this process can be observed in modern media environments all along; individuals grow in their compulsive seeking for rewards and develop increasingly irrational habits in the pursuit of social approval. The habits of curating their online personas have been described before; and the extents to which the representations differ from their lived reality can reach downright absurd levels. The experiences I witnessed throughout the years that I worked with teenagers, of whom virtually every individual had their online persona, could only confirm the statements I cited from peer works earlier. Interestingly, the portrayal of an accomplished, beautiful, wealthy or else socially desirable individual would not remain static but rather grow along the expectations of the audience. That is, in order to achieve validation steadily, the next posts would need more, *of everything*. How this is bound to end in a massive mental downward spiral needs no further explanation.

The copncept of instant gratification relates closely to the behavioral patterns explained. According to Bickel & Marsch (2001), instant gratification is the desire for immediate reward (i.e. pleasure), without delay or effort. It reflects the human tendency to prefer smaller and therefore immediate rewards over larger, but delayed ones, often linked to the dopaminergic pathways. It is a fundamental aspect in impulse control and has great relevance in the observations around social validation and digital social behavior. When individuals receive social validation, phasic dopamine spikes and thereby reinforces the performed action (Schultz, 1998), which means, that the brain forms an association between pleasure and the preference for immediate reward. While serotonin is the critical counterweight in this dynamic, its long-term depletion makes the individual less capable to get out of the cycle that starts to form, even if the short-term pleasure conflicts with long-term goals (Carver et al., 2008). Low serotonin, high dopamine states make the brain hyper-responsive to instant gratification with a significantly diminished control – this closes the gap to compulsion (Boureau & Dayan, 2011; Valkenburg & Peter, 2011). As described before, it is exactly the kind of behavior, that taps into the mechanisms of social networks, because they foster prolonged activity with their services and ultimately translate into more advertising revenue. The large-scale dysregulation in individuals is collateral damage.

The last aspect I want to mention here is the consequence of a deteriorated serotonin system after the surge in dopamine fades. In inevitable crash phases, and when validation is not provided, absent or withheld, the compromised serotonin system is too depleted to offer emotional resilience, guarding the individual against what would necessarily follow: anxiety and depression. In the absence of new rewards, there is a lack of psychological stabilizer, opening the door for heightened distress. As we now know, this is the exact same foundation, that compulsive actions have. They are meant to relieve this inner tension, even though irrational or ill-fitted, and even though they may exacerbate the underlying problem. At this point, individuals are too vulnerable to shield the temptations of getting deeper into the spiral, by perhaps enhancing their online presence, or do whatever they feel they need to do in order to get the craved-for stimulus. While at the same time, they live in distorted realities inward *and* outward, meaning they perceive themselves as irrationally inferior, and others as irrationally *superior*, there is a dual reinforcement at play. Not only are they, in state of their validation withdrawal, presented with the seeming perfection that others live, but also the inferiority complex is nourished by the consequences of their weakened rationalizing emotional stabilizer serotonin. This means anxiety and depression kick in open doors.

A growing body of evidence supports the strong correlations between modern social media use and mental health problems, especially regarding different forms of social anxieties, depression and obsessive-compulsive disorders, oftentimes in a state of co-morbidity. While the correlations between online behavior and mental health could easily fill a standalone book, I only want to highlight some of the most seminal examples at this point, that support the points I raised.

While high consumption rates of social media tend to correlate with susceptibility for depression (Ivie et al., 2020; Radovic et al., 2017; Kelly et al., 2018; Azem et al., 2023; Thoridottir et al., 2019), there seems to be a bi-directional relationship indicating that depressive symptoms can in turn increase social media use (Heffer et al., 2019). Considering the fact, that depressed individuals tend to isolate themselves more and avoid social situations, it may explain their heightened dependency on digital media. Shannon et al. (2021) confirmed, that the poor mental health state in individuals with high social media activity can be traced back to online validation patterns. Low self-esteem, poor image of one's own body and frequent upwards comparison have been reported numerous times, in numerous studies, and seem to especially affect young girls (Puukko et al., 2020; Kelly et al., 2018; Radovic et al., 2017). Unsurprisingly, exactly the same applies to social anxieties. Especially less resilient individuals have been recommended high caution in the frequent use of social media, as a comparative analysis of more than 1,700 studies highlighted (Lopes et al., 2022). We can derive from that information that the triangular correlation between low serotonin levels, high social media activity and poor mental health with high prevalence of anxious symptoms stand in close relation to each other. Regarding the numbers, assuming coincidence is hardly possible. Furthermore, 'problematic' social media use, as termed by Coyne et al. (2020) was found in direct correlation with anxiety disorders, particularly concerning the phenomenon of social comparison. Worsley et al. (2018) found similar results, concluding that attachment anxieties and problematic social media use correlated strongly. Regarding the pathology of obsessive compulsive disorder, the establishment is more difficult, since on the one hand, the act of engaging with social media, from our perspective, equals the compulsion itself, and on the other hand, the character of the disease can be highly diverse. Nevertheless, Aladwani & Al-Marzouq (2016) describe the reinforcing character of online platforms, particularly Facebook (which was in 2016, when Instagram was less popular and Tik Tok did not exist yet!), closely resemble the patterns observed in OCD, characterizing the permanent checking of mobile devices as an act that can be described as compulsive. Tan et al. (2020) and Sentürk et al. (2021) found, that the intermittent rewards provided on social media platforms are the mechanisms that reinforce behavioral patterns just like perpetuation of OCD rituals. While Tan et al.'s study was focused on peer groups for OCD in social media, one of the contributing factors of negative experiences was social comparison. Sentürk et al. (2021) term the obsessive use *addiction*.

7 NEUROADAPTATION TO MODERN 'ACHIEVEMENT CULTURE' AND ITS IMPLICATIONS FOR ADLER'S INFERIORITY CONCEPT

Aside from representing curated personas in digital networks, our modern culture has placed a specific emphasis on individual status and success for some time. Especially professional success and the hierarchical standing in their profession is an important source of self-confidence for most individuals nowadays. Performance is an indicator for self-worth and also for the perception of other people. Low-performers are perceived at least with pity, while high-performers are often regarded with envy and admiration. Dweck (1999) states in his work on achievement culture, that the self-worth derived from performance and achievement has an internalizing effect on people, creating their own framework for valuation, in which failure is stigmatized and personal value is directly linked to meeting certain standards. Obviously, the reinforcement of inadequacy is not far fetched in this framework. In a society, where achievement is the primary determinant of self-worth, individuals may easily develop an inferiority complex. This applies especially because achievement culture has its own means of entrenching this way of thinking and *feeling*. Since achievement is permanently displayed, and is expected to be displayed, individuals are not only constantly confronted with others' achievements, but have an innate pressure to display their own. Through heavy reliance on status symbols it is easy to tell apart the apparent high-performers from the low-performers. Through that, achievement culture induces not only inferiority complexes but also drives the desire to overcome it. On the other hand, given its dynamics, it contributes to compulsive attempts (Kirkpatrick & Ellis, 2001).

Linking back to Festinger (1954), it becomes obvious, how even early findings in social psychology laid the groundworks for our modern understanding of how these tie together: the clear tendency for upwards comparison is the main individual ground for the perpetuated experience of falling short; since success, performance and status are the main variables of comparison, today more present than ever, our natural wiring is practically *made* to walk into this trap. Moreover, today, what we see is often not real – easily intensifying the perceived gap between oneself and one's aspirations (Vogel et al., 2014). It is, however, strongly dependent on the culture an indidivual grows up and learns in. As Bandura's (1977) social learning theory posits, individuals are strongly bound to learn from their immediate environments and thus adopt the cultural knowledge and thinking. Triandis (1995) found, accordingly, that cultures that place a high emphasis on achievement and competition render individuals in a state of constant self-evaluation; which, as we have just pieced together will inevitably conclude '*not good enough*'. The human brain now has its own ways to react to constant reinforcement of these beliefs: pressure and expectation entrench themselves in our thinking, our belief systems and lastly, through neuroplasticity, in our behavior. We obtain dopamine hits from validation, that tells us, we belong and we are doing well. These neuroadaptations however are a powerful trap, as they cause our brain to overemphasize dopamine and rely on permanent stimulation of dopamine pathways – a compulsion develops (Schultz, 2007); reinforcing the neurological association between self-worth and validation from external sources. Over time, our brain does not only adapt to these beliefs, but it will also develop undesired reactions to withdrawal or absence of these validating stimuli: as serotonin gradually depletes, it can no more balance and smooth out the permanent spikes in the dopaminergic system, leading to the typical range of symptoms associated with low serotonin levels. In turn, the symptomy in the low serotonin pathology align accurately with the correlations observed in problematic social media use.

In addition, chronic stress from anxious behavioral patterns and depressed symptoms may stem from the fear of failure to meet societal expectations, since we reinforce these in ourselves through our reward-seeking patterns. This may lead to changes in the *hypothalamic-pituitary-adrenal (HPA)* axis and influence cortisol release, upon which we react with emotional dysregulation, particularly anxiety. This is due to the negative influence in specific brain areas responsible for decision-making and regulation of fear and impulsive emotions, in particular the amygdala and the prefrontal cortex (McEwen, 2007). This stress response, in turn, fuels the cycle again, leading to more signaling to seeking to overcome our inferiority, avoid societal rejection, and so forth.

8 THE UNIFICATION OF PERSPECTIVES

This chapter aims to guide through and eventually synthesize the key elements discussed in the previous sections and present the conclusions we have reached in a cohesive manner. It will outline the reasoning and connections between the points previously raised. Engaging with the material covered thus far, along with the extensive literature provided, has been a significant investment of time and may have posed various challenges. Therefore, I find it particularly rewarding to now assemble these insights into a unified perspective, reflecting on the journey from beginning to end and finally piece all sections together.

The Evolution, Amplification and Consequences of Modern Social Validation

Human beings have evolved as inherently social beings, with their survival historically linked to group cohesion and mutual support. In early societies, the pursuit of social acceptance and validation was crucial for ensuring access to resources, protection, and successful reproduction. As a result, group dynamics and collective norms emerged as mechanisms to maintain cohesion, leading to the development of early social structures and hierarchies where individuals derived their identity and status from their functional contributions to the group. Identity however, was not characterized by the depth of reflection as we know it, since the tribe and its survival and maintenance were prioritized over individual personality. This evolutionary foundation established a complex relationship between social behavior and neurochemical processes, influencing the trajectory of human development.

From Evolution to Modern Society: Transformation of Validation Mechanisms

As human societies gradually expanded and evolved, so too did the mechanisms for social validation. Early tribal systems, which were primarily focused on very basic needs, gradually evolved into more complex societal structures where identity and status became increasingly linked to achievements beyond mere survival. Throughout the transition from tribal to agricultural, and ultimately industrial, societies introduced new dimensions of social validation, including the accumulation of wealth, professional success, and subsequently, the emergence of status symbols such as material possessions. With the evolution into materialism, the public display of status became increasingly prevalent and salient. These transformations were not only social in nature but also closely connected to human neurobiology. Dopamine-driven reward systems, originally developed to reinforce survival behaviors, and embedded deeply into the genetic makeup, began to adapt – or in some cases, struggle to adapt – to the broader and more complex social frameworks. The brain's reward circuitry, including the Ventral Tegmental Area (VTA), Nucleus Accumbens (NAc), and Prefrontal Cortex (PFC), continued to respond to validation stimuli but now faced increasingly complex forms of social achievement and recognition, that misaligned with stimulus inputs known from previous eras. Slowly but surely, the pace at which society evolved and neurobiological structures failed to adapt in real-time, began to take up.

Status Symbols and the Neurochemical Shift

The emergence of status symbols during the industrial era, characterized by wealth accumulation and conspicuous consumption, has significantly and sustainably impacted human behavior. The pursuit of material success became a means of social validation, thereby reinforcing activities that conform to societal achievement standards. As advertising and media advanced, they effectively engaged the brain's reward system by associating status symbols with the neurochemical rewards the human brain had always been wired to pursue. These marketing strategies have played a crucial role in establishing social norms and creating aspirational ideals, consistently stimulating the brain's reward pathways by promising social acceptance and approval through material possessions and creating storytelling narratives of living a better life through purchasing and identifying with brands and brand ambassadors. This evolution has contributed to the internalization of social standards that extend beyond basic survival, encompassing societal achievement, success, and particularly ideals of bodily perfection. Consequently, individuals' self-worth has increasingly become linked to external validation, whether through wealth, status, or accomplishments, starting to heighten the potential for psychological stress. The human brain, which developed within the context of smaller, simpler social environments, was now confronted with the intricate complexities of modern social expectations and the innate threat of inadequacy.

The Digital Era: Amplification of Evolutionary Tendencies and Neurochemical Dysregulation

The digital age, particularly through the emergence and stark rise of social media, has significantly enhanced these evolutionary trends. Social networks have broadened the scope of social validation from localized and immediate contexts to a global and ubiquitous scale, and at an amazing pace. This meant yet another fundamental transformation of the nature and speed of social feedback, and by far the most substantial, yet in the shortest of the observed timeframes. What had previously evolved within millenials, and subsequently at least a few centuries, was now getting close to realtime; overwhelming human evolution. Platforms such as Instagram, Twitter, and Facebook have introduced real-time metrics of validation – such as likes, shares, and followers – which offer immediate and quantifiable social feedback. More than that; the metrics at public display have become a means of status themselves, not only resembling a numeric real-time terminal for one's social standing, but also a means of showcasing popularity (or *un*popularity) to the outside world. The brain's dopamine pathways, evolved over millennia to seek social approval for survival, are now often overwhelmed by a continuous influx of digital responses. Each instance of digital approval stimulates dopamine release, reinforcing behaviors and fostering the desire for further validation. In contrast to early human societies, where validation was infrequent and closely linked to survival, contemporary digital environments supply an ongoing stream of social comparison and feedback, leading to a cyclical pattern of dopamine-driven behavior.

Neurochemical Imbalance: Dopamine, Serotonin, and the Compulsive Feedback Loop

The overactivation of the brain's reward system, driven by the continuous pursuit of social validation online, results in an imbalance between dopamine and serotonin. Dopamine plays a key role in the anticipation and reception of rewards, while serotonin is essential for regulating mood and emotional stability. Excessive stimulation from digital feedback mechanisms can deplete serotonin levels, leading to mood instability, anxiety, and increased vulnerability to depressive states. The relationship between dopamine and serotonin is vital and delicate; as dopamine levels rise in response to online validation, serotonin may not adequately stabilize the emotional response, resulting in emotional fluctuations similar to those observed in affective disorders. When the brain becomes overstimulated by dopamine, it tends to desensitize over time, necessitating greater and more frequent validation to achieve the same level of satisfaction. This phenomenon mirrors patterns seen in substance addiction, while the consequences mirror bipolar behavior to an extent. The rush of a dopamine hit, in anticipation of a reward, is followed by a crash, that over time, can no more be smoothed out by a healthy serotonin balance. Consequently, this neurochemical imbalance fosters compulsive behaviors, where individuals become locked in a cycle of seeking validation, experiencing momentary emotional highs, and facing emotional lows in the absence of feedback or when receiving negative responses. The strain on mental health is high, since the loop is extremely difficult to control and to escape.

The Modern Inferiority Complex and Achievement Culture

Alfred Adler's theory of the inferiority complex is crucial for comprehending the psychological impacts of modern societal dynamics. In today's environment, the pressure to achieve success is closely linked to the incessant opportunity for social comparison facilitated by digital media, and virtually inescapable for most individuals – especially teenagers and young adults. Individuals now compare themselves not only to their immediate peers but also to a curated, global standard of excellence. Social media platforms amplify the tendency for upward comparisons, presenting idealized images of success, beauty, and lifestyle that are often unrealistic. This is not a coincidence; the companies behind social networks operate on advertising revenue that is closely linked to the time users spend on their apps. Consequently, algorithms carefully curate the contents displayed to each user, irrespective of the potential harm they may cause. This continuous exposure to idealized benchmarks intensifies feelings of inadequacy (we may add, that in users who have not yet found their 'place' in life, and are still in development of their identity, are particularly susceptible to being influenced and discouraged, suffering from insecurities as a natural part of growing up), thereby reinforcing the inferiority complex as individuals perceive themselves as consistently falling short. The compulsive nature of upward comparison and the internalization of these unattainable ideals compel individuals to establish increasingly unrealistic expectations for themselves, frequently resulting in perfectionistic tendencies and a relentless pursuit of achievement to counter perceived inferiority. However, these standards remain unachievable for the majority, leading to a persistent cycle of seeking validation and experiencing failure, which further contributes to anxiety, depression, and compulsive behaviors. A growing body of evidence substantiates these observations.

Neurochemical Insights: Persistent Dysregulation and Cognitive Overload

The continuous quest for validation, coupled with the associated neurochemical responses, can result in long-term disruptions in cognitive and emotional regulation. Social media platforms, by offering constant feedback and metrics for social approval, may overwhelm the brain's ability to process social information effectively. Historically, the human brain has evolved to manage stable, smaller social groups, as indicated by Dunbar's number. However, modern digital environments flood individuals with an overwhelming number of social connections and feedback, leading to cognitive overload. This makes it increasingly challenging for individuals to navigate the extensive array of social interactions and expectations. Furthermore, the ongoing overactivation of the dopamine system, without sufficient modulation from serotonin, can lead to neurochemical fatigue. As serotonin levels decrease, individuals may experience ongoing mood fluctuations, anxiety, and depressive symptoms, potentially resulting in chronic mental health challenges. This neurochemical imbalance, combined with a compulsive desire for validation to help stabilize mood and selfesteem, fosters a feedback loop that can be difficult to break. As we must mention at this point, research on the highly complex nuances and balances in the dopamine and serotonin circuitry, with partial overlaps in pathways, actions and reactions, is still subject to research to this day; yet, all we know about the brains involved regions and circuitries strongly points in the direction that we are right in these conclusions.

The Role of Cognitive Reinforcement and Neuroadaptation

Variable reinforcement schedules, which are integral to the functioning of social media algorithms, play a significant role in sustaining user engagement. The unpredictable nature of social feedback, akin to the principles of operant conditioning first described by Skinner and based on the findings by Pavlov in the early and mid 20th century, encourages users to seek continual affirmation, thereby fostering an addictive (or addiction-*like*) cycle. This dynamic resembles patterns seen in gamblingor substance addiction, where the anticipation of rewards often outweighs the rewards themselves and where the reward is sought after even in spite of full awareness over the detriment of the entire action. As time progresses, the brain adapts to this cycle, leading to an increased tolerance that necessitates higher levels of social feedback to elicit the same feelings of satisfaction, known as tolerance, and induced by desensitization of receptors for the reward-neurotransmitters released. This process of adaptation deepens the reliance on social approval and can lead to a decrease in serotonin levels in favor of dopamine due to the brain's essential 'rewiring' – where the dopamine circuitry takes precedence over serotonin in the brain – resulting in a chronic state of neurochemical imbalance. The ongoing quest for validation and achievement to counteract feelings of inadequacy may evolve into a compulsive pattern, echoing obsessive-compulsive behaviors. This, in turn, can contribute to a cycle of anxiety, depression, and emotional distress; on the one hand because serotonin fails to balance out the over-stimulated dopamine-reliant brain circuitry, and on the other hand because the focus in the psychological self is centered around own shortcomings and the own gravitation towards overcoming own feelings of inferiority.

9 CONCLUSION AND OUTLOOK PERSONAL EXPERIENCES FROM CLIENT-FOCUSED ENVIRONMENTS

In conclusion, the exploration of social validation from tribal societies to modern digital age highlights a fundamental aspect of human nature: our intrinsic need for belonging, acceptance, and affirmation. What originated as an evolutionary necessity for survival has transformed into a multifaceted array of behaviors influenced by cultural, technological, and neurochemical factors. This transition has not only increased the pressure to achieve and conform but has also significantly impacted our self-perception and the way we view others and our environments. For many, the quest for digital approval has become compulsive, influenced by neurochemical pathways that were originally adapted for simpler social environments.

Nonetheless, this narrative is not solely one of loss or imbalance. Acknowledging the challenges present in our digital society presents opportunities for growth and adaptation. By understanding the factors that drive our behaviors and recognizing the distortions imposed by modern media on our perceptions, individuals can begin to regain control over their mental and emotional health. The pivotal aspect is awareness: developing mindfulness regarding the influence of social platforms on our self-image and learning to distinguish between digital facades and authentic self-worth. The path ahead requires a thoughtful reassessment of our habits and belief systems. It calls for stepping back from the continuous engagement with social media and reconnecting with our values and desires independent of external validation. Insights from individuals who have successfully navigated this environment indicate that through mindful engagement, cognitive restructuring, and intentional behavior modifications, it is possible to foster a healthier relationship with ourselves and with the technology that surrounds us. Ultimately, the objective is not to entirely dismiss validation or achievement, but to pursue it in ways that are consistent with our authentic and intrinsic values. This journey towards self-acceptance and resilience against societal pressures is not about rejecting the pursuit of excellence; rather, it aims to redefine achievement in a manner that enhances our well-being rather than detracting from it. The challenge lies in striking a balance - acknowledging our evolutionary foundations while adjusting our minds and practices to meet the demands of the modern world, yet without a *make it or fake it*-attitude.

In my pertaining work in diverse settings, with burned out and depressed individuals in professional rehabilitation, and in media-centered counseling and mental health consultation for both adults and teenagers and their parents, I work with combinations of approaches to achieve improvements on different levels. Those integrate client-centered strategies, with elements from Cognitive Behavioral Therapy (CBT), psychoeducation and awareness, media literacy and to a large extent, metacognitive psychology. While the results are continually encouraging, this is neither a quantitative nor a qualitative research report; rather, it shares insights regarding how combinations of these strategies assist clients in developing more awareness and subsequently, mindful adaptations or their perceptions and behavioral patterns. The incorporation of metacognitive psychology focuses on enhancing clients' awareness of their own thought processes and patterns and the influence of these thoughts on their emotional responses and behaviors. Through that, individuals gain a reflective distance from their habits and are enabled to take an observing perspective on their own mental processes. It is however not without challenges, as the ability for metacognition is linked to overall intelligence and thus, the depth and timeframe vary. Metacognitive perspectives are particularly valuable when addressing the pervasive effects of social media and guiding clients towards an awareness of their automatic and mostly distorted perceptions arising from digital interactions. Clients learn to observe their thinking habits and recognize these inner automatisms, most importantly the internalization of unrealistic standards, automatic upwards comparisons and validation-seeking. In an ideal scenario, these realizations go along with the individual beginning to question the validity of these thoughts and recognizing the impact on their life. Psychoeducation can help them become aware of the relationships between cognitive filtering and reinforcement mechanisms, albeit broken down to their absolute essentials as to not overwhelm. It is crucial to remember, that in those scenarios, individuals do already suffer from a very high cognitive load. Often, in clarifying how media fosters internalizations of the portrayed idealization as normative, the acknowledgement of own interpretations happens automatically.

I see it as important to strike a balance between these concepts and inferiority (complexes), since after all, media-induced suffering may only tap into existing inferiority issues and it is important not to spike random needles into a client's psyche and overwhelm them by throwing them into mental spirals. Staying closely with the feelings of being subpar in comparison to unrealistic standards portrayed by social media shall rather be an element of psychoeducation and not psychotherapy at this point. Therefore, carefully selecting elements from CBT is a useful technique to challenge these exact cognitive distortions and the connected thought patterns. While this progresses, clientcentered approaches in developing self-compassion and empathy has proven relatively easy most of the time.

I may suggest that individuals tend to develop a blaming attitude towards social media and therefore have an easier time in becoming more self-compassionate, but to be honest, I see little harm in blaming abstract algorithm-based online networks, that have indeed proven to pose toxic threats to mental health. After all, if it helps individuals to deal better with their compulsions and develop more self-compassion, it is for the better, if it goes without a radicalization of thoughts.

In developing critical awareness, it allows clients to take a step back and evaluate their consumption habits (i.e. dopamine-driven reward-seeking) and subsequently, establish mindful boundaries that are put in place as mental health guardrails. Engaging in more mindful consumption is not meant to refrain from social or digital media, but rather to detach from the deeply ingrained patterns, that, as we learned earlier, happen unconsciusly most of the time. Upon setting better boundaries, clients regularly report feeling more in control and less overwhelmed; some even opt to take total breaks from their online presence without explicit encouragement. An observation I have made frequently is that after careful psychoeducation, and upon realization of the true impact of these dynamics, individuals feel encouraged to do their own research on the 'toxicity' of the same. While we must carefully remind them not to fall prey to misinformation (again), it is often coupled with deep insights about own behavioral adjustments that they have made over a long time and in response to the stimuli they had been subjected to, over and over again. From my experience, this is the realization that fosters the most change. Again, we do not want to radicalize clients against social media; we are still *client*-centered. However, the deep insights about how they have gradually shifted their perspectives about themselves, in comparison to the standards portrayed by curated profiles, happens to be a turning point for many individuals I have talked to. In this case, we can expect sustainable change.

One last thing I would like to highlight is the work with

younger clients and especially teenagers. We must keep in mind, that depending on their age, they have mostly or entirely grown up in digital environments and to them, there is no more experience-based comparison possible with a life and a world without these online personas. Thus, many if not most of those individuals have integrated social media into their identity from a young age, which rises the stakes of engagement. In these cases, there is much more of en educational element, and more emphasis on psychoeducation, before elements of CBT can start to take effect. Gradual psychoeducation and the careful and slow introduction of metacognitive strategies shall foster awareness, but with the caution not to overwhelm. In young clients, cultivating an understanding of how their perceptions and behavior are largely shaped by the consumption of media goes slowly and steadily and needs to keep in mind the much lower tendency of those clients to be willing to cut back on their online presence. This is understandable, because to them, this is much more life-changing and substantial than to the formerly mentioned clients. That is not only because of their own lives and the substantial integration of digital devices and platforms, but also those of their peers. Thus, to them, cutting back might feel equal to dropping out of society and their peer circles. Despite these complexities, an integrated approach to healthier habits and gradually developing science-based insights is no less important for younger generations; on the contrary. Anchored in metacognitive awareness, guiding them to a more critical evaluation of the contents they consume and encouraging better selfregulation fosters changes that many clients report as significantly beneficial to their mental wellbeing.

References

Abidin, C. (2016). "Aren't these just young, rich women doing vain things online?" Influencer selfies as subversive frivolity. Social Media+ Society, 2(2), 1-17.

Abidin, C. (2016). Visibility labour: Engaging with influencers' fashion brands and #OOTD advertorial campaigns on Instagram. Media International Australia, 161(1), 86-100.

Abramowitz J. S. (2006). The psychological treatment of obsessive-compulsive disorder. Canadian journal of psychiatry. Revue canadienne de psychiatrie, 51(7), 407-416.

Abramowitz, J. S., Khandker, M., Nelson, C. A., Deacon, B. J., & Rygwall, R. (2006). The role of cognitive factors in the pathogenesis of obsessive-compulsive symptoms: a prospective study. Behaviour research and therapy, 44(9), 1361-1374.

Adler, A. (1925). The Practice and Theory of Individual Psychology. (P. Radin, Trans.). Kegan Paul, Trench, Trubner & Co.

Adler, A. (1927). Understanding Human Nature. Greenberg.

Adler, A. (1929). The Science of Living. George Allen & Unwin Ltd.

Adler, A. (1964). The Individual Psychology of Alfred Adler: A Systematic Presentation in Selections From His Writings. (H. L. Ansbacher & R. R. Ansbacher, Eds.). (Original work published 1956).

Adler, A. (1997). Understanding Life: An Introduction to the Psychology of Alfred Adler (C. Brett, Trans.). Oneworld.

(Original work published 1927).

Adler, A. (1999). Problems of Neurosis: A Book of Case-Histories (P. Mairet, Trans.). Routledge. (Original work published 1929).

Adler, A. (2009). Social Interest: Adler's Key to the Meaning of Life. (J. Linton & R. Vaughn, Trans.; C. Brett, Ed.). Oneworld. (Original work published 1933).

Adler, A. (2011). What Life Should Mean to You. (H. Stein, Trans., A. Porter, Ed.). Alfred Adler Institute of Northwestern Washington. (Original work published 1931).

Adler, A. (2013). The Case of Miss R.: The Interpretation of a Life Story. (E. Jensen & F. Jensen, Trans.). Routledge. (Original work published 1929).

Aiello, L. C., & Wheeler, P. (1995). The expensive-tissue hypothesis: The brain and the digestive system in human and primate evolution. Current Anthropology, 36(2), 199-221.

Aksoy-Aksel, A., Gall, A., Seewald, A., Ferraguti, F., & Ehrlich, I. (2021). Midbrain dopaminergic inputs gate amygdala intercalated cell clusters by distinct and cooperative mechanisms in male mice. eLife, 10, e63708.

Al-Hasani, R., Gowrishankar, R., Schmitz, G. P., et al. (2021). Ventral tegmental area GABAergic inhibition of cholinergic interneurons in the ventral nucleus accumbens shell promotes reward reinforcement. Nature Neuroscience.

Al-Hasani, R., Gowrishankar, R., Schmitz, G. P., Pedersen, C. E., Marcus, D. J., Shirley, S. E., Hobbs, T. E., Elerding, A. J., Renaud, S. J., Jing, M., Li, Y., Alvarez, V. A., Lemos, J. C., & Bruchas, M. R. (2021). Ventral tegmental area GABAergic inhibition of cholinergic interneurons in the ventral nucleus accumbens shell promotes reward reinforcement. Nature neuroscience, 24(10), 1414-1428.

Aladwani, A. M., & Almarzouq, M. (2016). Understanding compulsive social media use: The premise of complementing self-conceptions mismatch with technology. Computers in Human Behavior, 60, 575-581.

Albin R. L. (2019). Complementary motivational roles of nigroaccumbens and nigrostriatal dopaminergic pathways.

Movement disorders: official journal of the Movement Disorder Society, 34(1), 45.

Alden, L. E., & Taylor, C. T. (2004). Interpersonal processes in social phobia. Clinical Psychology Review, 24(7), 857-882.

Alex, K. D., & Pehek, E. A. (2007). Pharmacologic mechanisms of serotonergic regulation of dopamine neurotransmission. Pharmacology & therapeutics, 113(2), 296-320.

Alex, K. D., Yavanian, G. J., McFarlane, H. G., Pluto, C. P., & Pehek, E. A. (2005). Modulation of dopamine release by striatal 5-HT2C receptors. Synapse (New York, N.Y.), 55(4), 242-251.

Alter, A. (2017). Irresistible: The rise of addictive technology and the business of keeping us hooked. Penguin Press.

Alvard, M. (2009). Kinship and Cooperation. Human Nature.

Aman, T. K., Shen, R. Y., & Haj-Dahmane, S. (2007). D2-like dopamine receptors depolarize dorsal raphe serotonin neurons through the activation of nonselective cationic conductance. The Journal of pharmacology and experimental therapeutics, 320(1), 376-385.

American Psychiatric Association (APA). (2013). Diagnostic and Statistical Manual of Mental Disorders (5th ed.). Washington, DC.

Angst J. (1986). The course of affective disorders. Psychopathology, 19 Suppl 2, 47-52.

Appel, H., Gerlach, A. L., Crusius, J. (2016). The interplay between Facebook use, social comparison, envy, and depression. Current Opinion in Psychology, 9, 44-49.

Aspinwall, L. G., & Taylor, S. E. (1993). Effects of social comparison direction, threat, and self-esteem on affect, self-evaluation, and expected success. Journal of Personality and Social Psychology, 64(5), 708-722.

Assadi, S. M., Yucel, M., & Pantelis, C. (2009). Dopamine modulates neural networks involved in effort-based decision-making. Neuroscience and Biobehavioral Reviews, 33(3), 383-393.

150

Assmann, J. (1997). Moses the Egyptian: The memory of Egypt in western monotheism. Harvard University Press.

Astrakas, L. G., Elbach, S., Giannopulu, I., Li, S., Benjafield, H., & Tzika, A. A. (2023). The role of ventral tegmental area in chronic stroke rehabilitation: an exploratory study. Frontiers in neurology, 14, 1270783.

Azem, L., Al Alwani, R., Lucas, A., Alsaadi, B., Njihia, G., Bibi, B., Alzubaidi, M., & Househ, M. (2023). Social Media Use and Depression in Adolescents: A Scoping Review. Behavioral sciences (Basel, Switzerland), 13(6), 475.

Bandura, A. (1977). Social learning theory. Prentice Hall.

Barkow, J. H. (1989). Darwin, sex, and status: Biological approaches to mind and culture. University of Toronto Press.

Baudrillard, J. (1998). The consumer society: Myths and structures. SAGE Publications.

Baulac, M., Verney, C., & Berger, B. (1986). Dopaminergic innervation of the parahippocampal and hippocampal regions in the rat. Revue neurologique.

Bauman, Z. (2007). Consuming life. Polity Press.

Beart, P. M., & McDonald, D. (1982). 5-Hydroxytryptamine and 5-hydroxytryptaminergic-dopaminergic interactions in the ventral tegmental area of rat brain. The Journal of pharmacy and pharmacology, 34(9), 591-593.

Bechara, A., Damasio, H., & Damasio, A. R. (2000). Emotion, decision making and the orbitofrontal cortex. Cerebral cortex (New York, N.Y. : 1991), 10(3), 295-307.

Beck, A. T. (1976). Cognitive therapy and the emotional disorders. International Universities Press.

Beck, A. T. (1990). Cognitive therapy of personality disorders. Guilford Press.

Beck, A. T., Emery, G., & Greenberg, R. L. (1985). Anxiety disorders and phobias: A cognitive perspective. Basic Books.

Beck, U. (1992). Risk society: Towards a new modernity. SAGE Publications.

Beer, J. S., & Hughes, B. L. (2010). Neural systems of social comparison and the "above-average" effect. NeuroImage,

49(3), 2671-2679.

Beer, J. S., Lombardo, M. V., & Bhanji, J. P. (2010). Roles of medial prefrontal cortex and orbitofrontal cortex in selfevaluation. Journal of cognitive neuroscience, 22(9), 2108-2119.

Beierle, F., Probst, T., Allemand, M. ., Zimmermann, J. ., Pryss, R. ., Neff, P. ., Schlee, W., Stieger, S., & Budimir, S. (2020). Frequency and Duration of Daily Smartphone Usage in Relation to Personality Traits. Digital Psychology, 1(1), 20-28.

Berg, K. A., Harvey, J. A., Spampinato, U., & Clarke, W. P. (2005). Physiological relevance of constitutive activity of 5-HT2A and 5-HT2C receptors. Trends in pharmacological sciences, 26(12), 625-630.

Berger, J. (1972). Ways of seeing. Penguin Books.

Berger, M., Gray, J. A., & Roth, B. L. (2009). The expanded biology of serotonin. Annual review of medicine, 60, 355-366.

Berridge, K. C. (2007). The debate over dopamine's role in reward: the case for incentive salience. Psychopharmacology (Berl) 191: 391-431.

Berridge, K. C., & Robinson, T. E. (1998). What is the role of dopamine in reward: hedonic impact, reward learning, or incentive salience?. Brain research. Brain research reviews, 28(3), 309-369.

Berryman, C., Ferguson, C. J., & Negy, C. (2018). Social media use and mental health among young adults. Psychiatric Quarterly, 89, 307-314.

Berumen, L. C., Rodríguez, A., Miledi, R., & García-Alcocer, G. (2012). Serotonin receptors in hippocampus. TheScientificWorldJournal, 2012, 823493.

Bickel, W. K., & Marsch, L. A. (2001). Toward a behavioral economic understanding of drug dependence: delay discounting processes. Addiction (Abingdon, England), 96(1), 73-86.

Billieux, J., Maurage, P., Lopez-Fernandez, O. et al. (2015). Can Disordered Mobile Phone Use Be Considered a Behavioral Addiction? An Update on Current Evidence and a Comprehensive Model for Future Research. Curr Addict Rep 2, 156-162.

Blatt, S. J. (1995). The destructiveness of perfectionism: Implications for the treatment of depression. American Psychologist, 50(12), 1003-1020.

Bligh-Glover, W., Kolli, T. N., Shapiro-Kulnane, L., Dilley, G. E., Friedman, L., Balraj, E., Rajkowska, G., & Stockmeier, C. A. (2000). The serotonin transporter in the midbrain of suicide victims with major depression. Biological psychiatry, 47(12), 1015-1024.

Boehm, C. (1999). Hierarchy in the forest: The evolution of egalitarian behavior. Harvard University Press.

Boehm, C. (2012). Moral origins: The evolution of virtue, altruism, and shame. Basic Books.

Borgkvist, A., Malmlöf, T., Feltmann, K., Lindskog, M., & Schilström, B. (2011). Dopamine in the hippocampus is cleared by the norepinephrine transporter. The international journal of neuropsychopharmacology.

Bouarab, C., Thompson, B., & Polter, A. M. (2019). VTA GABA Neurons at the Interface of Stress and Reward. Frontiers in neural circuits, 13,78 .

Boureau, Y., & Dayan, P. (2011). Opponency Revisited: Competition and Cooperation Between Dopamine and Serotonin. Neuropsychopharmacology, 36, 74-97.

Bowlby, J. (1969). Attachment and loss: Vol. 1. Attachment. Basic Books.

Boyd, D. (2014). It's complicated: The social lives of networked teens. Yale University Press.

Boyd, D. M., & Ellison, N. B. (2007). Social network sites: Definition, history, and scholarship. Journal of ComputerMediated Communication, 13(1), 210-230.

Boyd, R., & Silk, J. B. (2018). How humans evolved. W.W. Norton & Company.

Brady C. F. (2014). Obsessive-compulsive disorder and common comorbidities. The Journal of clinical psychiatry, 75(1), e02.

Breward, C. (1995). The culture of fashion: A new history of fashionable dress. Manchester University Press.

Bruin, J. D. (1990). Orbital prefrontal cortex, dopamine, and social-agonistic behavior of male Long Evans rats. Aggressive Behavior, 16(3/4), 231-248.

Bubar, M. J., Stutz, S. J., & Cunningham, K. A. (2011). 5-HT(2C) receptors localize to dopamine and GABA neurons in the rat mesoaccumbens pathway. PloS one, 6(6), e20508.

Bucher, T. (2012). Want to be on the top? Algorithmic power and the threat of invisibility on Facebook. New Media & Society, 14(7), 1164-1180.

Bush, G., Luu, P., & Posner, M. I. (2000). Cognitive and emotional influences in anterior cingulate cortex. Trends in Cognitive Sciences, 4(6), 215-222.

Buunk, B. P., & Ybema, J. F. (1997). Social comparison and occupational stress: The identification-contrast model. In B. P. Buunk & F. X. Gibbons (Eds.), Health, coping, and well-being: Perspectives from social comparison theory (pp. 359-388). Erlbaum.

Buunk, B., Kuyper, H., van der Zee, Y. G. (2005). Affective response to social comparison in the classroom. Basic and Applied Social Psychology, 27, 229-237.

Cai, J., & Tong, Q. (2022). Anatomy and Function of Ventral Tegmental Area Glutamate Neurons. Frontiers in neural circuits, 16,867053 .

Canli, T., & Lesch, K. P. (2007). Long story short: the serotonin transporter in emotion regulation and social cognition. Nature neuroscience, 10(9), 1103-1109.

Carr, D. B., & Sesack, S. R. (2000). Projections from the rat prefrontal cortex to the ventral tegmental area: Target specificity in the synaptic associations with mesoaccumbens and mesocortical neurons. The Journal of Neuroscience.

Carr, N. (2010). The shallows: What the internet is doing to our brains. W.W. Norton & Company.

Carver, C. S., Johnson, S. L., & Joormann, J. (2008). Serotonergic function, two-mode models of self-regulation, and vulnerability to depression: what depression has in common with impulsive aggression. Psychological bulletin, 134(6), 912-943.

Caspi, A., Sugden, K., Moffitt, T. E., Taylor, A., Craig, I. W., Harrington, H., McClay, J., Mill, J., Martin, J., Braithwaite, A., & Poulton, R. (2003). Influence of life stress on depression: moderation by a polymorphism in the 5HTT gene. Science (New York, N.Y.), 301(5631), 386-389.

Castells, M. (2010). The rise of the network society. Wiley-Blackwell.

Catania A. C. (1973). Self-inhibiting effects of reinforcement. Journal of the experimental analysis of behavior, 19(3), 517-526.

Catania, A. C., & Reynolds, G. S. (1968). A quantitative analysis of the responding maintained by interval schedules of reinforcement. Journal of the Experimental Analysis of Behavior, 11(3), 327-383.

Celada, P., Puig, M. V., & Artigas, F. (2013). Serotonin modulation of cortical neurons and networks. Frontiers in integrative neuroscience, 7,25 .

Cetin, T., Freudenberg, F., Füchtemeier, M., & Koch, M. (2004). Dopamine in the orbitofrontal cortex regulates operant responding under a progressive ratio of reinforcement in rats. Neuroscience Letters, 370, 114-117.

Chau, B. K. H., Jarvis, H., Law, C. K., & Chong, T. T. (2018). Dopamine and reward: a view from the prefrontal cortex. Behavioural pharmacology, 29(7), 569-583.

Chou, H. T. G., & Edge, N. (2012). "They are happier and having better lives than I am": The impact of using Facebook on perceptions of others' lives. Cyberpsychology, Behavior, and Social Networking, 15(2), 117-121.

Claassen, D. O., Stark, A. J., Spears, C. A., Petersen, K. J., van Wouwe, N. C., Kessler, R. M., Zald, D. H., & Donahue, M. J. (2017). Mesocorticolimbic hemodynamic response in Parkinson's disease patients with compulsive behaviors. Movement disorders : official journal of the Movement Disorder Society, 32(11), 1574-1583.

Clark, D. M., & Wells, A. (1995). A cognitive model

of social phobia. In R. G. Heimberg (Ed.), Social phobia: Diagnosis, assessment, and treatment (pp. 69-93). Guilford Press.

Clarke, R., & Adermark, L. (2015). Dopaminergic Regulation of Striatal Interneurons in Reward and Addiction: Focus on Alcohol. Neural plasticity, 2015, 814567.

Clutton-Brock, T. H. (1974). Primate social organization and ecology. Nature, 250(5467), 539-542.

Coccaro E. F. (1989). Central serotonin and impulsive aggression. The British journal of psychiatry. Supplement, (8), 52-62.

Collins, R. (1996). For better or worse: The impact of upward social comparison on self-evaluations. Psychological Bulletin, 119, 51-69.

Collins, R. L. (1996). For better or worse: The impact of upward social comparison on self-evaluations. Psychological Bulletin, 119(1), 51-69.

Coppen A. (1967). The biochemistry of affective disorders. The British journal of psychiatry : the journal of mental science, 113(504), 1237-1264.

Coppen, A. J., & Doogan, D. P. (1988). Serotonin and its place in the pathogenesis of depression. The Journal of clinical psychiatry, 49 Suppl, 4-11.

Cortes, P. M., Hernández-Arteaga, E., Sotelo-Tapia, C., et al. (2019). Effects of inactivation of the ventral tegmental area on prefronto-accumbens activity and sexual motivation in male rats. Physiology & Behavior.

Cowen P. J. (1993). Serotonin receptor subtypes in depression: evidence from studies in neuroendocrine regulation. Clinical neuropharmacology, 16 Suppl 3, S6-S18.

Coyne, S. M., Rogers, A. A., Zurcher, J. D., Stockdale, L., & Booth, M. (2020). Does Time Spent Using Social Media Impact Mental Health? An Eight Year Longitudinal Study. Computers in Human Behavior, 104, Article ID: 106160.

Crawford, K. (2015). The anxieties of big data. The New Inquiry, 5(30), 1-13.

Crocker, J., & Luhtanen, R. K. (1990). Collective self-esteem and in-group bias. Journal of Personality and Social Psychology, 58(1), 60-67.

Crockett, M. J., Clark, L., Apergis-Schoute, A. M., Morein-Zamir, S., & Robbins, T. W. (2012). Serotonin modulates the effects of Pavlovian aversive predictions on response vigor. Neuropsychopharmacology : official publication of the American College of Neuropsychopharmacology, 37(10), 2244-2252.

Dalley, J. W., Mar, A. C., Economidou, D., & Robbins, T. W. (2008). Neurobehavioral mechanisms of impulsivity: fronto-striatal systems and functional neurochemistry. Pharmacology, biochemistry, and behavior, 90(2), 250-260.

Dalley, J. W., Theobald, D. E., Eagle, D. M., Passetti, F., & Robbins, T. W. (2002). Deficits in impulse control associated with tonically-elevated serotonergic function in rat prefrontal cortex. Neuropsychopharmacology : official publication of the American College of Neuropsychopharmacology, 26(6), 716-728.

Davies, G. (1996). A history of money: From ancient times to the present day. University of Wales Press.

Dayan P. (2009). Dopamine, reinforcement learning, and addiction. Pharmacopsychiatry, 42 Suppl 1, S56-S65.

De Botton, A. (2004). Status anxiety. Pantheon Books.

De Deurwaerdère, P., & Spampinato, U. (1999). Role of serotonin(2A) and serotonin(2B/2C) receptor subtypes in the control of accumbal and striatal dopamine release elicited in vivo by dorsal raphe nucleus electrical stimulation. Journal of neurochemistry, 73(3), 1033-1042.

De Deurwaerdère, P., Navailles, S., Berg, K. A., Clarke, W. P., & Spampinato, U. (2004). Constitutive activity of the serotonin2C receptor inhibits in vivo dopamine release in the rat striatum and nucleus accumbens. The Journal of neuroscience : the official journal of the Society for Neuroscience, 24(13), 3235-3241.

Deci, E. L., & Ryan, R. M. (1985). Intrinsic motivation and self-determination in human behavior. Plenum.

Del Arco, A., & Mora, F. (2009). Neurotransmitters and prefrontal cortex-limbic system interactions: Implications for plasticity and psychiatric disorders. Journal of Neural Transmission.

Di Giovanni, G., De Deurwaerdére, P., Di Mascio, M., Di Matteo, V., Esposito, E., & Spampinato, U. (1999). Selective blockade of serotonin-2C/2B receptors enhances mesolimbic and mesostriatal dopaminergic function: a combined in vivo electrophysiological and microdialysis study. Neuroscience, 91(2), 587-597.

Di Matteo, V., Di Giovanni, G., Pierucci, M., & Esposito, E. (2008). Serotonin control of central dopaminergic function: focus on in vivo microdialysis studies. Progress in brain research, 172, 7-44.

Dixon, M. L., Thiruchselvam, R., Todd, R., & Christoff, K. (2017). Emotion and the prefrontal cortex: An integrative review. Psychological bulletin, 143(10), 1033-1081.

Douglas, M., & Isherwood, B. (1979). The World of Goods. Norton.

Duman, R. S., & Aghajanian, G. K. (2012). Synaptic dysfunction in depression: potential therapeutic targets. Science (New York, N.Y.), 338(6103), 68-72.

Duman, R. S., Aghajanian, G. K., Sanacora, G., & Krystal, J. H. (2016). Synaptic plasticity and depression: new insights from stress and rapid-acting antidepressants. Nature medicine, 22(3), 238-249.

Dumas, T. M., Maxwell-Smith, M. A., Davis, J. P., & Giulietti, P. A. (2017). Lying or longing for likes? Narcissism, peer belonging, loneliness and normative versus deceptive like-seeking on Instagram in emerging adulthood. Computers in Human Behavior, 71, 1-10.

Dunbar, R. I. M. (1992). Neocortex size as a constraint on group size in primates. Journal of Human Evolution, 22(6), 469-493.

Dunbar, R. I. M. (1993). Coevolution of neocortex size, group size, and language in humans. Behavioral and Brain Sciences, 16(4), 681-694.

Dunbar, R. I. M. (1996). Grooming, gossip, and the evolution of language. Harvard University Press.

Dunnett, S. B., Bunch, S. T., Gage, F. H., & Björklund, A. (1984). Dopamine-rich transplants in rats with 6-OHDA lesions of the ventral tegmental area. I. Effects on spontaneous and drug-induced locomotor activity. Behavioural Brain Research.

Durkheim, E. (1893). The Division of Labour in Society. New York: The Free Press.

Durkheim, É. (1912). The elementary forms of religious life. George Allen & Unwin.

Duvarci, S., & Pare, D. (2014). Amygdala microcircuits controlling learned fear. Neuron, 82(5), 966-980.

Dweck, C. S. (1999). Self-theories: Their role in motivation, personality, and development. Psychology Press.

Dwortz, M. F., Curley, J. P., Tye, K. M., & Padilla-Coreano, N. (2022). Neural systems that facilitate the representation of social rank. Philosophical transactions of the Royal Society of London. Series B, Biological sciences, 377 (1845), 20200444.

Eberhard, V., Matthes, S. A., Ulrich, J. (2015). The need for social approval and the choice of gender-typed occupations. Journal of Gender Studies.

Edwards, D. H., & Kravitz, E. A. (1997). Serotonin, social status and aggression. Current opinion in neurobiology, 7(6), 812-819.

Ehrlich, I., Humeau, Y., Grenier, F., Ciocchi, S., Herry, C., & Lüthi, A. (2009). Amygdala inhibitory circuits and the control of fear memory. Neuron, 62(6), 757-771.

Elhai, J. D., Levine, J. C., Dvorak, R. D., & Hall, B. J. (2017). Non-Social Features of Smartphone Use are Most Related to Depression, Anxiety and Problematic Smartphone Use. Computers in Human Behavior, 69, 75-82.

Eliade, M. (1958). Rites and symbols of initiation. Harper & Row.

Elliott, R., & Deakin, B. (2005). Role of the orbitofrontal cortex in reinforcement processing and inhibitory control: evidence from functional magnetic resonance imaging studies in healthy human subjects. International Review of Neurobiology, 65, 89-116.

Ellis, A. (1962). Reason and emotion in psychotherapy. Lyle Stuart.

Ellison, N. B., Heino, R., & Gibbs, J. (2006). Managing impressions online: Self-presentation processes in the online dating environment. Journal of Computer-Mediated Communication, 11(2), 415-441.

Ellison, N. B., Steinfield, C., & Lampe, C. (2007). The benefits of Facebook "friends:" Social capital and college students' use of online social network sites. Journal of Computer-Mediated Communication, 12(4), 1143-1168.

Euston, D. R., Gruber, A. J., & McNaughton, B. L. (2012). The role of medial prefrontal cortex in memory consolidation. Annual Review of Neuroscience.

Ewen, S. (1976). Captains of consciousness: Advertising and the social roots of the consumer culture. McGraw-Hill.

Fardouly, J., Diedrichs, P. C., Vartanian, L. R., & Halliwell, E. (2015). Social comparisons on social media: The impact of Facebook on young women's body image concerns and mood. Body Image, 13, 38-45.

Fareri, D. S., & Delgado, M. R. (2014). Social Rewards and Social Networks in the Human Brain. The Neuroscientist : a review journal bringing neurobiology, neurology and psychiatry, 20(4), 387-402.

Farmer, C. M., Klauer, S. G., McClafferty, J. A., & Guo, F. (2015). Secondary Behavior of Drivers on Cell Phones. Traffic injury prevention, 16(8), 801-808.

Feist, J., & Feist, G. J. (2008). Theories of personality (7th ed.). McGraw-Hill.

Ferenczi, E. A., Zalocusky, K. A., Liston, C., Grosenick, L., Warden, M. R., Amatya, D., Katovich, K., Mehta, H., Patenaude, B., Ramakrishnan, C., Kalanithi, P., Etkin, A., Knutson, B., Glover, G. H., & Deisseroth, K. (2016). Prefrontal cortical regulation of brainwide circuit dynamics and reward-related behavior. Science (New York, N.Y.), 351(6268), aac 9698.

Ferster, C. B., & Skinner, B. F. (1957). Schedules of reinforcement. Appleton-Century-Crofts.

Festinger, L. (1954). A theory of social comparison processes. Human Relations, 7(2), 117-140.

Festinger, L. (1957). A theory of cognitive dissonance. Stanford University Press.

Fiorillo, C. D., Tobler, P. N., & Schultz, W. (2003). Discrete coding of reward probability and uncertainty by dopamine neurons. Science (New York, N.Y.), 299(5614), 1898-1902.

Fiorino, D. F., Coury, A., Fibiger, H. C., & Phillips, A. G. (1993). Electrical stimulation of reward sites in the ventral tegmental area increases dopamine transmission in the nucleus accumbens of the rat. Behavioural brain research, 55(2), 131-141.

Firat, A. F., & Venkatesh, A. (1995). Liberatory postmodernism and the reenchantment of consumption. Journal of Consumer Research, 22(3), 239-267.

FitzGerald, T. H. B., Seymour, B., & Dolan, R. (2009). The Role of Human Orbitofrontal Cortex in Value Comparison for Incommensurable Objects. The Journal of Neuroscience, 29, 8388-8395.

Flannery, K. V. (1972). The cultural evolution of civilizations. Annual Review of Ecology and Systematics, 3(1), 399-426.

Flannery, K., & Marcus, J. (2012). The creation of inequality: How our prehistoric ancestors set the stage for monarchy, slavery, and empire. Harvard University Press.

Fletcher, P. J., Tampakeras, M., Sinyard, J., & Higgins, G. A. (2007). Opposing effects of 5-HT(2A) and 5-HT(2C) receptor antagonists in the rat and mouse on premature responding in the five-choice serial reaction time test. Psychopharmacology, 195(2), 223-234.

Fliessbach, K., Weber, B., Trautner, P., Dohmen, T., Sunde, U., Elger, C. E., & Falk, A. (2007). Social comparison affects reward-related brain activity in the human ventral striatum. Science, 318(5854), 1305-1308.

Flink, J. J. (1975). The car culture. MIT Press.

Foddy, M., & Crundall, I. (1993). A field study of social

comparison processes in ability evaluation. British Journal of Social Psychology, 32(4), 287-305.

Foley, R. (2002). Adaptive radiations and dispersals in hominin evolutionary ecology. Evolutionary Anthropology: Issues, News, and Reviews, 11(2), 32-37.

Foley, R. A., & Lee, P. C. (1989). Finite social space, evolutionary pathways, and reconstructing hominid behavior. Science, 243(4893), 901-906.

Frank, T. (1997). The conquest of cool: Business culture, counterculture, and the rise of hip consumerism. University of Chicago Press.

Franz, B. (2014). What you don't know can hurt you: Social comparison on Facebook. Thesis; Ohio State University.

Freud, A. (1936). The ego and the mechanisms of defense. International Universities Press.

Fried, M. H. (1967). The evolution of political society: An essay in political anthropology. Random House.

Frith, K., Shaw, P., & Cheng, H. (2005). The construction of beauty: A cross-cultural analysis of women's magazine advertising. Journal of Communication, 55(1), 56-70.

Frost, R. O., & Steketee, G. (Eds.). (2002). Cognitive approaches to obsessions and compulsions: Theory, assessment, and treatment. Pergamon/Elsevier Science Inc.

Fudge, J. L., & Emiliano, A. B. (2003). The extended amygdala and the dopamine system: Another piece of the dopamine puzzle. The Journal of Neuropsychiatry and Clinical Neurosciences, 15(3), 306-316.

Fudge, J. L., & Emiliano, A. B. (2003). The extended amygdala and the dopamine system: another piece of the dopamine puzzle. The Journal of neuropsychiatry and clinical neurosciences, 15(3), 306-316.

Fukuyama, F. (2011). The origins of political order: From prehuman times to the French Revolution. Farrar, Straus and Giroux.

Gamble, C. (1999). The palaeolithic societies of Europe. Cambridge University Press.

Gangarossa, G., Longueville, S., De Bundel, D., Perroy, J.,

Hervé, D., Girault, J., & Valjent, E. (2012). Characterization of dopamine D1 and D2 receptor-expressing neurons in the mouse hippocampus. Hippocampus.

Gao, S. H., Shen, L. L., Wen, H. Z., Zhao, Y. D., Chen, P. H., & Ruan, H. Z. (2020). The projections from the anterior cingulate cortex to the nucleus accumbens and ventral tegmental area contribute to neuropathic pain-evoked aversion in rats. Neurobiology of disease, 140, 104862.

Gasbarri, A., Sulli, A., & Packard, M. (1997). The dopaminergic mesencephalic projections to the hippocampal formation in the rat. Progress in Neuro-Psychopharmacology and Biological Psychiatry.

Gaze, E. (2023). Eric Gaze Debunks the Dunning-Kruger Effect. Bowdoin College. Retrieved from: http://www.bowdoin.edu/news/2023/05/eric-gaze-debunks-dunning-kruger-effect.html

Gerlitz, C., & Helmond, A. (2013). The like economy: Social buttons and the data-intensive web. New Media & Society, 15(8), 1348-1365.

Giddens, A. (1990). The consequences of modernity. Stanford University Press.

Gilbert, P. (2016). Depression: The Evolution of Powerlessness (1st ed.). Routledge

Gilbert, P., & Irons, C. (2009). Shame, self-criticism, and self-compassion in adolescence. In N. Allen & L. Sheeber (Eds.), Adolescent emotional development and the emergence of depressive disorders (pp. 195-214). Cambridge University Press.

Gillespie, T. (2014). The relevance of algorithms. In T. Gillespie, P. Boczkowski, & K. Foot (Eds.), Media technologies: Essays on communication, materiality, and society (pp. 167-194). MIT Press.

Gillespie, T. (2018). Custodians of the internet: Platforms, content moderation, and the hidden decisions that shape social media. Yale University Press.

Gillihan, S. J., Rao, H., Wang, J., Detre, J. A., Breland, J., Sankoorikal, G. M., Brodkin, E. S., & Farah, M. J. (2010).

Serotonin transporter genotype modulates amygdala activity during mood regulation. Social cognitive and affective neuroscience, 5(1), 1-10.

Gilovich, T., Kumar, A., & Jampol, L. (2015). A wonderful life: Experiential consumption and the pursuit of happiness. Journal of Consumer Psychology, 25(1), 152-165.

Gobert, A., Rivet, J. M., Lejeune, F., Newman-Tancredi, A., Adhumeau-Auclair, A., Nicolas, J. P., Cistarelli, L., Melon, C., & Millan, M. J. (2000). Serotonin(2C) receptors tonically suppress the activity of mesocortical dopaminergic and adrenergic, but not serotonergic, pathways: a combined dialysis and electrophysiological analysis in the rat. Synapse (New York, N.Y.), 36(3), 205-221.

Goedhoop, J., Arbab, T., & Willuhn, I. (2023). Anticipation of Appetitive Operant Action Induces Sustained Dopamine Release in the Nucleus Accumbens. The Journal of neuroscience : the official journal of the Society for Neuroscience, 43(21), 3922-3932.

Goffman, E. (1959). The presentation of self in everyday life. Doubleday Anchor.

Goldman, R., & Papson, S. (1996). Sign wars: The cluttered landscape of advertising. Guilford Press.

Gonzales, R. A., & Weiss, F. (1998). Suppression of ethanol-reinforced behavior by naltrexone is associated with attenuation of the ethanol-induced increase in dialysate dopamine levels in the nucleus accumbens. The Journal of neuroscience : the official journal of the Society for Neuroscience, 18(24), 10663-10671.

Goodman, W. K., Price, L. H., Rasmussen, S. A., Mazure, C., Fleischmann, R. L., Hill, C. L., Heninger, G. R., & Charney, D. S. (1989). The Yale-Brown Obsessive Compulsive Scale. I. Development, use, and reliability. Archives of general psychiatry, 46(11), 1006-1011.

Grace, A. (2000). The Tonic / Phasic Model of Dopamine System Regulation and its Implications for Understanding Alcohol and Psychostimulant Craving. Addiction, 95(2): 119-128.

Graeber, D. (2011). Debt: The first 5000 years. Melville House.

Grant, J. E., & Phillips, K. A. (2005). Recognizing and treating body dysmorphic disorder. Annals of clinical psychiatry : official journal of the American Academy of Clinical Psychiatrists, 17(4), 205-210.

Grimm, O., Nägele, M., Küpper-Tetzel, L., de Greck, M., Plichta, M., & Reif, A. (2021). No effect of a dopaminergic modulation fMRI task by amisulpride and L-DOPA on reward anticipation in healthy volunteers. Psychopharmacology, 238(5), 1333-1342.

Groenewegen, H.J., Voorn, P., Scheel-Krüger, J. (2016). Limbic-Basal Ganglia Circuits Parallel and Integrative Aspects. In: Soghomonian, JJ. (Eds.). The Basal Ganglia. Innovations in Cognitive Neuroscience. Springer, Cham.

Groman, S. M., et al. (2013). Monoamine levels within the orbitofrontal cortex and putamen interact to predict reversal learning performance. Biological Psychiatry.

Gross, T. (2023). Handbook for Higher Education. Vol. 1, Sociodynamics and the Theory of Mind: Scientific Foundations and Principles in Language Proficiency and Communication.

Gross, T. (2023). The Socio-economy of Surveillance Capitalism in the Context of User Cognition and Psychology. IJASE., 11(02): 157-170.

Gross, T. (2024). Cognitive Nemesis: A Psychological Synthesis. Minkowski Institute Press.

Gross, T., Michaud, A., Zerrouki, Y., & Hamood, A. (2024). Debunking Instagram's Algorithm Sugarcoating. (ZeMV e-Publikation, 05/2024). Zentrum für Medienpsychologie und Verhaltensforschung.

Gruninger T. R., LeBoeuf B., Liu Y., Garcia, L. R. (2007). Molecular signaling involved in regulating feeding and other motivated behaviors. Mol Neurobiol 35: 1-20.

Guan, X. M., & McBride, W. J. (1989). Serotonin microinfusion into the ventral tegmental area increases accumbens dopamine release. Brain research bulletin, 23(6), 541-

547.

Gurven, M., & Hill, K. (2009). Why do men hunt? A reevaluation of "Man the Hunter" and the sexual division of labor. Current Anthropology, 50(1), 51-74.

Haber, S. N. (2011). Neuroanatomy of Reward: A View from the Ventral Striatum. In: Gottfried J. A. (Ed.). Neurobiology of Sensation and Reward, 11. Taylor & Francis.

Habermas, J. (1989). The structural transformation of the public sphere: An inquiry into a category of bourgeois society. MIT Press.

Hamilton, W. D. (1964). The genetical evolution of social behaviour. I. Journal of Theoretical Biology, 7(1), 1-16.

Hansen, K. B., Yi, F., Perszyk, R. E., Furukawa, H., Wollmuth, L. P., Gibb, A. J., & Traynelis, S. F. (2018). Structure, function, and allosteric modulation of NMDA receptors. The Journal of general physiology, 150(8), 1081-1105.

Harada, M., Pascoli, V., Hiver, A., Flakowski, J., & Lüscher, C. (2021). Corticostriatal Activity Driving Compulsive Reward Seeking. Biological psychiatry, 90(12), 808-818.

Harmer C. J. (2008). Serotonin and emotional processing: does it help explain antidepressant drug action?. Neuropharmacology, 55(6), 1023-1028.

Harmer, C. J., Mackay, C. E., Reid, C. B., Cowen, P. J., & Goodwin, G. M. (2006). Antidepressant drug treatment modifies the neural processing of nonconscious threat cues. Biological psychiatry, 59(9), 816-820.

Hart, D., & Sussman, R. W. (2005). Man the hunted: Primates, predators, and human evolution. Westview Press.

Harter, S. (1983). Developmental perspectives on the self-system. In P. H. Mussen (Ed.), Handbook of child psychology (Vol. 4, pp. 275-385). Wiley.

Heatherton, T. F. (2011). Neuroscience of self and self-regulation. Annual Review of Psychology, 62, 363-390.

Heffer, T., Good, M., Daly, O., MacDonell, E., & Willoughby, T. (2019). The longitudinal association between socialmedia use and depressive symptoms among adolescents and young adults: An empirical reply to Twenge et al. (2018).

Clinical Psychological Science, 7(3), 462-470.

Heimberg, R. G., Liebowitz, M. R., Hope, D. A., & Schneier, F. R. (2010). Social phobia: Diagnosis, assessment, and treatment. Guilford Press.

Henrich, J., & Gil-White, F. J. (2001). The evolution of prestige: Freely conferred deference as a mechanism for enhancing the benefits of cultural transmission. Evolution and Human Behavior, 22(3), 165-196.

Higgins, G. A., & Fletcher, P. J. (2003). Serotonin and drug reward: focus on 5-HT2C receptors. European journal of pharmacology, 480(1-3), 151-162.

Higley, J. D., Suomi, S. J., & Linnoila, M. (1996). A non-human primate model of type II alcoholism? Part 2. Diminished social competence and excessive aggression correlates with low cerebrospinal fluid 5hydroxyindoleacetic acid concentrations. Alcoholism, clinical and experimental research, 20(4), 643-650.

Hill, R. A., & Dunbar, R. I. M. (2003). Social network size in humans. Human Nature, 14(1), 53-72.

Hirano, K., Kimura, R., Sugimoto, Y., Yamada, J., Uchida, S., Kato, Y., Hashimoto, H., & Yamada, S. (2005). Relationship between brain serotonin transporter binding, plasma concentration and behavioural effect of selective serotonin reuptake inhibitors. British journal of pharmacology, 144(5), 695-702.

Hitchcott, P. K., Bonardi, C., & Phillips, G. D. (1997). Enhanced stimulus-reward learning by intra-amygdala administration of a D3 dopamine receptor agonist. Psychopharmacology, 133(3), 240-248.

Hobbes, T. (1651). Leviathan. Andrew Crooke.

Hobsbawm, E. (1968). Industry and empire: From 1750 to the present day. Penguin Books.

Hogan, B. (2010). The presentation of self in the age of social media: Distinguishing performances and exhibitions online. Bulletin of Science, Technology & Society, 30(6), 377-386.

Holt, D. B. (2002). Why do brands cause trouble? A

dialectical theory of consumer culture and branding. Journal of Consumer Research, 29(1), 70-90.

Horney, K. (1937). The neurotic personality of our time. W.W. Norton & Company.

Horvitz J. C. (2002). Dopamine gating of glutamatergic sensorimotor and incentive motivational input signals to the striatum. Behavioural brain research, 137(1-2), 65-74

Hrdy, S. B. (2009). Mothers and others: The evolutionary origins of mutual understanding. Harvard University Press.

Hu, E., & Nguyen, A. (2022). Too Much Pleasure Can Lead to Addiction. How To Break the Cycle and Find a Balance. NPR. Retrieved from: https://www.npr.org/2022/03/31/1090009509/addiction-how-to-break-the-cycle-and-find-balance

Huidobro-Toro, J. P., Valenzuela, C. F., & Harris, R. A. (1996). Modulation of GABAA receptor function by G protein-coupled 5-HT2C receptors. Neuropharmacology, 35(9-10), 1355-1363.

Hull, C. L. (1943). Principles of Behavior. Appleton-Century-Crofts.

Humphrey, N. (1976). The social function of intellect. In P. P. G. Bateson & R. A. Hinde (Eds.), Growing points in ethology (pp. 303-317). Cambridge University Press.

Humphries, M. D., & Prescott, T. J. (2010). The ventral basal ganglia, a selection mechanism at the crossroads of space, strategy, and reward. Progress in neurobiology, 90(4), 385-417.

Isaac, G. L. (1978). The food-sharing behavior of proto-human hominids. Scientific American, 238(4), 90-108.

Ivie, E. J., Pettitt, A., Moses, L. J., & Allen, N. B. (2020). A meta-analysis of the association between adolescent social media use and depressive symptoms. Journal of affective disorders, 275, 165-174.

Jackson, K. T. (1985). Crabgrass frontier: The suburbanization of the United States. Oxford University Press.

Jefferies-Sewell, K., Chamberlain, S. R., Fineberg, N. A., & Laws, K. R. (2017). Cognitive dysfunction in body dysmorphic disorder: new implications for nosological systems and neurobiological models. CNS spectrums, 22(1), 51-60.

Jenkins, T. A., Nguyen, J. C., Polglaze, K. E., & Bertrand, P. P. (2016). Influence of Tryptophan and Serotonin on Mood and Cognition with a Possible Role of the Gut-Brain Axis. Nutrients, 8(1), 56.

Jhally, S. (1987). The codes of advertising: Fetishism and the political economy of meaning in the consumer society. Routledge.

Johnson, A. W., & Earle, T. (1987). The evolution of human societies: From foraging group to agrarian state. Stanford University Press.

Johnson, A. W., & Earle, T. (2000). The evolution of human societies: From foraging group to agrarian state. Stanford University Press.

Johnson, C. S., Stapel, D. (2010). Harnessing social comparisons: When and how upward comparisons influence goal pursuit. Basic and Applied Social Psychology, 32, 234-242.

Joiner, T. E., Jr, Brown, J. S., & Wingate, L. R. (2005). The psychology and neurobiology of suicidal behavior. Annual review of psychology, 56, 287-314.

Jung, C. G. (1954). The development of personality. Princeton University Press.

Jung, W. H., & Kim, H. (2020). Intrinsic functional and structural brain connectivity in humans predicts individual social comparison orientation. Frontiers in Psychiatry.

Kaplan, H., Hill, K., Lancaster, J., & Hurtado, A. M. (2000). A theory of human life history evolution: Diet, intelligence, and longevity. Evolutionary Anthropology: Issues, News, and Reviews, 9(4), 156-185.

Keath, J. R., Iacoviello, M. P., Barrett, L. E., Mansvelder, H. D., & McGehee, D. S. (2007). Differential modulation by nicotine of substantia nigra versus ventral tegmental area dopamine neurons. Journal of neurophysiology, 98(6), 3388-3396.

Kedia, G., Mussweiler, T., & Linden, D. E. (2014). Brain mechanisms of social comparison and their influence on the reward system. Neuroreport, 25(16), 1255-1265.

Kelly, R. L. (1995). The foraging spectrum: Diversity in hunter-gatherer lifeways. Smithsonian Institution Press.

Kelly, Y., Zilanawala, A., Booker, C., & Sacker, A. (2019). Social Media Use and Adolescent Mental Health: Findings From the UK Millennium Cohort Study. EClinicalMedicine, 6, 59-68.

Kemp, A. H., Gray, M. A., Silberstein, R. B., Armstrong, S. M., & Nathan, P. J. (2004). Augmentation of serotonin enhances pleasant and suppresses unpleasant cortical electrophysiological responses to visual emotional stimuli in humans. NeuroImage, 22(3), 1084-1096.

Kernberg, O. F. (1975). Borderline conditions and pathological narcissism. Jason Aronson.

Khayat, A., & Yaka, R. (2024). Activation of nucleus accumbens projections to the ventral tegmental area alters molecular signaling and neurotransmission in the reward system. Frontiers in Molecular Neuroscience.

Kienast, T., Hariri, A. R., Schlagenhauf, F., Wrase, J., Sterzer, P., Buchholz, H. G., Smolka, M. N., Gründer, G., Cumming, P., Kumakura, Y., Bartenstein, P., Dolan, R. J., & Heinz, A. (2008). Dopamine in amygdala gates limbic processing of aversive stimuli in humans. Nature neuroscience, 11(12), 1381-1382.

Kim, D., Kim, J., & Kim, H. (2023). Distinctive Roles of Medial Prefrontal Cortex Subregions in Strategic Conformity to Social Hierarchy. The Journal of neuroscience : the official journal of the Society for Neuroscience, 43(36), 6330-6341.

Kim, S. W., Park, S. Y., & Hwang, O. (2002). Up-regulation of tryptophan hydroxylase expression and serotonin synthesis by sertraline. Molecular pharmacology, 61(4), 778-785.

King R. (2002). Cognitive therapy of depression. Aaon Beck, John Rush, Brian Shaw, Gary Emery. New York: Guilford, 1979. The Australian and New Zealand journal of psychiatry, 36(2), 272-275.

Kirkpatrick, L. A., & Ellis, B. J. (2004). An Evolutionary-

Psychological Approach to Self-esteem: Multiple Domains and Multiple Functions. In M. B. Brewer & M. Hewstone (Eds.), Self and social identity (pp. 52-77). Blackwell Publishing.

Kiser, D., SteemerS, B., Branchi, I., & Homberg, J. R. (2012). The reciprocal interaction between serotonin and social behaviour. Neuroscience and Biobehavioral Reviews, 36(2), 786-798.

Kleemans, M., Daalmans, S., Carbaat, I., & Anschütz, D. J. (2018). Picture perfect: The direct effect of manipulated Instagram photos on body image in adolescent girls. Media Psychology, 21(1), 93-110.

Klein, N. (2000). No logo: Taking aim at the brand bullies. Picador.

Knauft, B. M. (1991). Violence and sociality in human evolution. Current Anthropology, 32(4), 391-428.

Kohlberg, L. (1981). Essays on moral development. Harper & Row.

Koob G. F. (2008). Hedonic Homeostatic Dysregulation as a Driver of Drug-Seeking Behavior. Drug discovery today. Disease models, 5(4), 207-215.

Koob, G. F., & Le Moal, M. (1997). Drug abuse: hedonic homeostatic dysregulation. Science (New York, N.Y.), 278(5335), 52-58.

Koob, G. F., & Le Moal, M. (2001). Drug addiction, dysregulation of reward, and allostasis. Neuropsychopharmacology : official publication of the American College of Neuropsychopharmacology, 24(2), 97129.

Koob, G. F., Buck, C. L., Cohen, A., Edwards, S., Park, P. E., Schlosburg, J. E., Schmeichel, B., Vendruscolo, L. F., Wade, C. L., Whitfield, T. W., Jr, & George, O. (2014). Addiction as a stress surfeit disorder. Neuropharmacology, 76 Pt B(0 0), 370-382.

Korb, S., Götzendorfer, S. J., Massaccesi, C., Sezen, P., Graf, I., Willeit, M., Eisenegger, C., & Silani, G. (2020). Dopaminergic and opioidergic regulation during anticipation and consumption of social and nonsocial rewards. eLife, 9 , e55797.

Koski, J. E., McHaney, J. R., Rigney, A. E., & Beer, J. S. (2020). Reconsidering longstanding assumptions about the role of medial prefrontal cortex (MPFC) in social evaluation. NeuroImage.

Koutlas, I., Patrikiou, L., van der Starre, S. E., et al. (2024). Distinct ventral tegmental area neuronal ensembles are indispensable for reward-driven approach and stress-driven avoidance behaviors. Preprint.

Krasnova, H., Wenninger, H., Widjaja, T., Buxmann, P. (2013). Envy on Facebook: A hidden threat to users' life satisfaction? Wirtschaftsinformatik, 92, 1-16.

Kringelbach, M. L., & Berridge, K. C. (2010). The Neuroscience of Happiness and Pleasure. Social research, 77(2), 659-678.

Kröner, S., Rosenkranz, J. A., Grace, A. A., & Barrionuevo, G. (2005). Dopamine modulates excitability of basolateral amygdala neurons in vitro. Journal of Neurophysiology, 93(3), 1598-1610.

Kross, E., Verduyn, P., Demiralp, E., Park, J., Lee, D. S., Lin, N., Shablack, H., Jonides, J., & Ybarra, O. (2013). Facebook use predicts declines in subjective well-being in young adults. PloS one, 8(8), e69841.

Kruger, J., & Dunning, D. (1999). Unskilled and unaware of it: How difficulties in recognizing one's own incompetence lead to inflated self-assessments. Journal of Personality and Social Psychology, 77(6), 1121-1134.

Kuhn R. (1958). The treatment of depressive states with G 22355 (imipramine hydrochloride). The American journal of psychiatry, 115(5), 459-464.

Kulikov, A. V., Gainetdinov, R. R., Ponimaskin, E., Kalueff, A. V., Naumenko, V. S., & Popova, N. K. (2018). Interplay between the key proteins of serotonin system in SSRI antidepressants efficacy. Expert opinion on therapeutic targets, 22(4), 319-330.

Lange, P. V. (2008). Social comparison is basic to social psychology. American Journal of Psychology, 124, 169-172.

Leary, M. R., Baumeister, R. F. (2000). The nature and function of self-esteem: Sociometer theory. Advances in Experimental Social Psychology, 32, 1-62.

Leaver, T., Highfield, T., & Abidin, C. (2020). Instagram: Visual social media cultures. Polity Press.

Lee, J. H., Lee, S., & Kim, J.-H. (2017). Amygdala circuits for fear memory: A key role for dopamine regulation. The Neuroscientist, 23(6), 542-553.

Lee, R. B., & Daly, R. (1999). The Cambridge encyclopedia of hunters and gatherers. Cambridge University Press.

Lee, R. B., & DeVore, I. (1968). Man the hunter. Aldine de Gruyter.

Leiss, W., Kline, S., & Jhally, S. (1986). Social communication in advertising: Persons, products and images of wellbeing. Methuen.

Leu-Semenescu, S., Arnulf, I., Decaix, C., Moussa, F., Clot, F., Boniol, C., Touitou, Y., Levy, R., Vidailhet, M., & Roze, E. (2010). Sleep and rhythm consequences of a genetically induced loss of serotonin. Sleep, 33(3), 307-314.

Lévi-Strauss, C. (1962). Totemism. Beacon Press.

Licinio, J., & Wong, M.- (2002). Brain-derived neurotrophic factor (BDNF) in stress and affective disorders. Molecular psychiatry, 7(6), 519.

Ling, Y., Gao, B., Jiang, B., Fu, C., & Zhang, J. (2023). Materialism and envy as mediators between upward social comparison on social network sites and online compulsive buying among college students. Frontiers in Psychology.

Linnoila, V. M., & Virkkunen, M. (1992). Aggression, suicidality, and serotonin. The Journal of clinical psychiatry, 53 Suppl, 46-51.

Liu, Z., Bunney, E. B., Appel, S. B., & Brodie, M. S. (2003). Serotonin reduces the hyperpolarization-activated current (Ih) in ventral tegmental area dopamine neurons: involvement of 5-HT2 receptors and protein kinase C. Journal of neurophysiology, 90(5), 3201-3212.

Lomborg, S. (2013). Social media, social genres: Making sense of the ordinary. Routledge.

Lopes, L. S., Valentini, J. P., Monteiro, T. H., Costacurta, M. C. F., Soares, L. O. N., Telfar-Barnard, L., & Nunes, P. V. (2022). Problematic Social Media Use and Its Relationship with Depression or Anxiety: A Systematic Review. Cyberpsychology, behavior and social networking, 25(11), 691-702.

Lovejoy, C. O. (1981). The origin of man. Science, 211 (4480), 341-350.

Lowry, C. A. (2002). Functional Subsets of Serotonergic Neurones: Implications for Control of the Hypothalamic-Pituitary-Adrenal Axis. Journal of Neuroendocrinology, 14 (11), 911-923.

Lu, J., Zhong, X., Liu, H., Hao, L., Huang, C. T., Sherafat, M. A., Jones, J., Ayala, M., Li, L., & Zhang, S. C. (2016). Generation of serotonin neurons from human pluripotent stem cells. Nature biotechnology, 34(1), 89-94.

Lucki I. (1998). The spectrum of behaviors influenced by serotonin. Biological psychiatry, 44(3), 151-162.

Luo, Y., Eickhoff, S. B., Hétu, S., & Feng, C. (2018). Social comparison in the brain: A coordinate-based metaanalysis of functional brain imaging studies on the downward and upward comparisons. Human Brain Mapping, 39(1), 440-458.

Magnus, J., & Peresetsky, A. (2022). A Statistical Explanation of the Dunning-Kruger Effect. Frontiers in Psychology, 13:840180.

Mandelli, L., Serretti, A., Marino, E., Pirovano, A., Calati, R., & Colombo, C. (2007). Interaction between serotonin transporter gene, catechol-O-methyltransferase gene and stressful life events in mood disorders. The international journal of neuropsychopharmacology, 10(4), 437-447.

Marchand, R. (1985). Advertising the American dream: Making way for modernity, 1920-1940. University of California Press.

Markus, H., & Wurf, E. (1987). The dynamic self-concept: A social psychological perspective. Annual Review of Psychology, 38(1), 299-337.

Marlowe, F. W. (2005). Hunter-gatherers and human evolution. Evolutionary Anthropology: Issues, News, and Reviews, 14(2), 54-67.

Marshall, P. D. (1997). Celebrity and power: Fame in contemporary culture. University of Minnesota Press.

Marwick, A. E. (2013). Status update: Celebrity, publicity, and branding in the social media age. Yale University Press.

Marwick, A. E., & Boyd, D. (2014). Networked privacy: How teenagers negotiate context in social media. New Media & Society, 16(7), 1051-1067.

Marwick, A., & Boyd, D. (2011). To see and be seen: Celebrity practice on Twitter. Convergence, 17(2), 139-158.

Maurizi C. P. (1990). The therapeutic potential for tryptophan and melatonin: possible roles in depression, sleep, Alzheimer's disease and abnormal aging. Medical hypotheses, 31(3), 233-242.

Mazur, J. E. (1986). Learning and behavior. Prentice Hall.

McAdams, D. P. (1993). The stories we live by: Personal myths and the making of the self. William Morrow.

McBride, W. J., Murphy, J. M., Lumeng, L., & Li, T. K. (1990). Serotonin, dopamine and GABA involvement in alcohol drinking of selectively bred rats. Alcohol (Fayetteville, N.Y.), 7(3), 199-205.

McEwen B. S. (2007). Physiology and neurobiology of stress and adaptation: central role of the brain. Physiological reviews, 87(3), 873-904.

McGaugh, J. L. (2002). Memory consolidation and the amygdala: A systems perspective. Trends in Neurosciences, 25(9), 456-461.

McKendrick, N., Brewer, J., & Plumb, J. H. (1982). The birth of a consumer society: The commercialization of eighteenth-century England. Indiana University Press.

Melaugh, S., & Cowlishaw, O. (2021). Algorithms, Social Media & Mass Manipulation. Ikario Podcast. Accessed from: https://ikario.com/033/

Meltzer H. Y. (1990). Role of serotonin in depression.

Annals of the New York Academy of Sciences, 600, 486-500.

Meltzer, H. Y., & Nash, J. F. (1988). Serotonin and Mood: Neuroendocrine Aspects. In: (D. Ganten, & D. Pfaff. (Eds.). Neuroendocinology of Mood. Springer.

Merens, W., Willem Van der Does, A. J., & Spinhoven, P. (2007). The effects of serotonin manipulations on emotional information processing and mood. Journal of affective disorders, 103(1-3), 43-62.

Meshi, D., Tamir, D. I., & Heekeren, H. R. (2015). The Emerging Neuroscience of Social Media. Trends in cognitive sciences, 19(12), 771-782.

Michely, J., Eldar, E., Martin, I. M., & Dolan, R. J. (2020). A mechanistic account of serotonin's impact on mood. Nature communications, 11(1), 2335.

Midgley, E. (2013). Keeping in Touch or Keeping Score? Social Comparisons on Facebook. Thesis; University of Toronto.

Millan, M. J., Dekeyne, A., & Gobert, A. (1998). Serotonin (5-HT)2C receptors tonically inhibit dopamine (DA) and noradrenaline (NA), but not 5-HT, release in the frontal cortex in vivo. Neuropharmacology, 37(7), 953-955.

Millan, M. J., Lejeune, F., & Gobert, A. (2000). Reciprocal autoreceptor and heteroreceptor control of serotonergic, dopaminergic and noradrenergic transmission in the frontal cortex: relevance to the actions of antidepressant agents. Journal of psychopharmacology (Oxford, England), 14(2), 114-138.

Mithen, S. (1996). The prehistory of the mind: A search for the origins of art, religion and science. Thames and Hudson.

Miyazaki, K. W., Miyazaki, K., Tanaka, K. F., Yamanaka, A., Takahashi, A., Tabuchi, S., & Doya, K. (2014). Optogenetic activation of dorsal raphe serotonin neurons enhances patience for future rewards. Current biology : CB , 24(17), 2033-2040.

Molenberghs, P., & Morrison, S. (2014). The role of the medial prefrontal cortex in social categorization. Social Cognitive and Affective Neuroscience, 9(3), 292-298.

Mongrain, M. (1998). Parental representations and support-seeking behaviors related to dependency and selfcriticism. Journal of Personality, 66(3), 151-173.

Montardy, Q., Zhou, Z., Lei, Z., Liu, X., Zeng, P., Chen, C., Liu, Y., Sanz-Leon, P., Huang, K., & Wang, L. (2019). Characterization of glutamatergic VTA neural population responses to aversive and rewarding conditioning in freelymoving mice. Science bulletin, 64(16), 1167-1178.

Morales, M., & Barbano, M. F. (2023). Midbrain (VTA) Circuits. In: Giplin, N. W. (Ed.). Neurocircuitry of Addiction, 45-72. Academic Press.

Morgan, T., Rendell, L., Ehn, M., Hoppitt, W., Laland, K. (2012). The evolutionary basis of human social learning. Proceedings of the Royal Society B: Biological Sciences, 279, 653-662.

Mosak, H. H., & Maniacci, M. P. (1999). A primer of Adlerian psychology: The analytic-behavioral-cognitive psychology of Alfred Adler. Routledge.

Müller, C. P., & Jacobs, B. L. (Eds.). (2010). Handbook of the behavioral neurobiology of serotonin. Elsevier Academic Press.

Mussweiler, T., Rüter, K., & Epstude, K. (2004). The ups and downs of social comparison: Mechanisms of assimilation and contrast. Journal of Personality and Social Psychology, 87(6), 832-844.

Nakao, T., Takezawa, T., Miyatani, M., & Ohira, H. (2009). Medial prefrontal cortex and cognitive regulation. Psychologia: An International Journal of Psychological Sciences, 52(2), 93-109.

Nakazato T. (2019). Dual-mode dopamine increases mediated by 5-HT1B and 5-HT2C receptors inhibition, inducing impulsive behavior in trained rats. Experimental brain research, 237(10), 2573-2584.

Narita, M., Matsushima, Y., Niikura, K., Narita, M., Takagi, S., Nakahara, K., Kurahashi, K., Abe, M., Saeki, M., Asato, M., Imai, S., Ikeda, K., Kuzumaki, N., & Suzuki, T. (2010). Implication of dopaminergic projection from the ventral tegmental area to the anterior cingulate cortex in μ-opioid-induced place preference. Addiction biology, 15(4), 434-447.

Narvaes, R., & Martins de Almeida, R. M. (2014). Aggressive behavior and three neurotransmitters: dopamine, GABA, and serotonin-A review of the last 10 years.Psychology & Neuroscience, 7(4), 601-607.

Navailles, S., Moison, D., Ryczko, D., & Spampinato, U. (2006). Region-dependent regulation of mesoaccumbens dopamine neurons in vivo by the constitutive activity of central serotonin2C receptors. Journal of neurochemistry, 99(4), 1311-1319.

Niederkofler, V., Asher, T. E., & Dymecki, S. M. (2015). Functional Interplay between Dopaminergic and Serotonergic Neuronal Systems during Development and Adulthood. ACS chemical neuroscience, 6(7), 1055-1070.

Nishi, A., Bibb, J. A., Snyder, G. L., Higashi, H., Nairn, A. C., & Greengard, P. (2000). Amplification of dopaminergic signaling by a positive feedback loop. Proceedings of the National Academy of Sciences of the United States of America, 97(23), 12840-12845.

Nomoto, K., Watanabe, T., & Sakagami, M. (2007). Dopamine Responses to Complex Reward-Predicting Stimuli. Neuroscience Research, 58.

Nugent, A. C., Carlson, P. J., Bain, E. E., Eckelman, W., Herscovitch, P., Manji, H., Zarate, C. A., Jr, & Drevets, W. C. (2013). Mood stabilizer treatment increases serotonin type 1A receptor binding in bipolar depression. Journal of psychopharmacology (Oxford, England), 27(10), 894-902.

Nuhfer, E. (2017). Collateral Metacognitive Damage. Online publication. Retrieved from http://www.improvewithmetacognition.com/collateral-metacognitivedamage/

Nutt, D. J., Ballenger, J. C., Sheehan, D., & Wittchen, H. U. (2002). Generalized anxiety disorder: comorbidity, comparative biology and treatment. The international journal of neuropsychopharmacology, 5(4), 315-325.

Oh, H., Piantadosi, S. C., Rocco, B. R., Lewis, D. A., Watkins, S. C., & Sibille, E. (2019). The Role of Dendritic Brain-Derived Neurotrophic Factor Transcripts on Altered Inhibitory Circuitry in Depression. Biological psychiatry, 85(6), 517-526.

Oulasvirta, A., Rattenbury, T., Ma, L. et al. (2012). Habits make smartphone use more pervasive. Pers Ubiquit Comput 16, 105-114.

Palmer, D., Cayton, C. A., Scott, A., Lin, I., Newell, B., Paulson, A., Weberg, M., & Richard, J. M. (2024). Ventral pallidum neurons projecting to the ventral tegmental area reinforce but do not invigorate reward-seeking behavior. Cell reports, 43(1), 113669 .

Parga, J., Rodriguez-Pallares, J., Muñoz, A., Guerra, M. J., & Labandeira-Garcia, J. L. (2007). Serotonin decreases generation of dopaminergic neurons from mesencephalic precursors via serotonin type 7 and type 4 receptors. Developmental neurobiology, 67(1), 10-22.

Park, Y. S., Sammartino, F., Young, N. A., Corrigan, J., Krishna, V., & Rezai, A. R. (2019). Anatomic Review of the Ventral Capsule/Ventral Striatum and the Nucleus Accumbens to Guide Target Selection for Deep Brain Stimulation for Obsessive-Compulsive Disorder. World neurosurgery, 126, 1-10.

Parker G. (2005). Beyond major depression. Psychological medicine, 35(4), 467-474.

Pascoli, V., Hiver, A., Van Zessen, R., Loureiro, M., Achargui, R., Harada, M., Flakowski, J., & Lüscher, C. (2018). Stochastic synaptic plasticity underlying compulsion in a model of addiction. Nature, 564(7736), 366-371.

Patodia, S., Somani, A., Liu, J., Cattaneo, A., Paradiso, B., Garcia, M., Othman, M., Diehl, B., Devinsky, O., Mills, J. D., Foong, J., & Thom, M. (2022). Serotonin transporter in the temporal lobe, hippocampus and amygdala in SUDEP. Brain pathology (Zurich, Switzerland), 32(5), e13074.

Pavlov, I. P. (1927). Conditioned Reflexes: An Investigation of the Physiological Activity of the Cerebral Cortex.

Oxford University Press.

Pazos, A., Probst, A., & Palacios, J. M. (1987). Serotonin receptors in the human brain–III. Autoradiographic mapping of serotonin-1 receptors. Neuroscience, 21(1), 97-122.

Pearce, E., & Moutsiou, T. (2014). Using obsidian transfer distances to explore social network maintenance in late Pleistocene hunter-gatherers. Journal of anthropological archaeology.

Pehek, E. A., & Hernan, A. E. (2015). Stimulation of glutamate receptors in the ventral tegmental area is necessary for serotonin-2 receptor-induced increases in mesocortical dopamine release. Neuroscience, 290, 159-164.

Pehek, E. A., Nocjar, C., Roth, B. L., Byrd, T. A., & Mabrouk, O. S. (2006). Evidence for the preferential involvement of 5-HT2A serotonin receptors in stress- and drug-induced dopamine release in the rat medial prefrontal cortex. Neuropsychopharmacology : official publication of the American College of Neuropsychopharmacology, 31(2), 265277.

Pellegrino, A. (2024). Social comparison, problems of digital consumption and its implications. In: Pellegrino, A. (2024). Decoding Digital Consumer Behavior. Springer.

Pempek, T. A., Yermolayeva, Y. A., & Calvert, S. L. (2009). College students' social networking experiences on Facebook. Journal of Applied Developmental Psychology, 30(3), 227-238.

Perez, S., & Lodge, D. (2018). Convergent Inputs from the Hippocampus and Thalamus to the Nucleus Accumbens Regulate Dopamine Neuron Activity. The Journal of Neuroscience.

Perugi, G., Akiskal, H. S., Pfanner, C., Presta, S., Gemignani, A., Milanfranchi, A., Lensi, P., Ravagli, S., & Cassano, G. B. (1997). The clinical impact of bipolar and unipolar affective comorbidity on obsessive-compulsive disorder. Journal of affective disorders, 46(1), 15-23.

Pew Research Center. (2018). Teens, social media & technology. Pew Research Center, Internet & Technology.

Pignatelli, M., & Bonci, A. (2015). Role of Dopamine

Neurons in Reward and Aversion: A Synaptic Plasticity Perspective. Neuron, 86(5), 1145-1157.

Polanyi, K. (1944). The great transformation: The political and economic origins of our time. Beacon Press.

Porras, G., Di Matteo, V., Fracasso, C., Lucas, G., De Deurwaerdère, P., Caccia, S., Esposito, E., & Spampinato, U. (2002). 5-HT2A and 5-HT2C/2B receptor subtypes modulate dopamine release induced in vivo by amphetamine and morphine in both the rat nucleus accumbens and striatum. Neuropsychopharmacology : official publication of the American College of Neuropsychopharmacology, 26(3), 311-324.

Pozzi, L., Acconcia, S., Ceglia, I., Invernizzi, R. W., & Samanin, R. (2002). Stimulation of 5-hydroxytryptamine (5HT2C)) receptors in the ventrotegmental area inhibits stress-induced but not basal dopamine release in the rat prefrontal cortex. Journal of neurochemistry, 82(1), 93-100.

Premack, D. (1965). Reinforcement Theory. In D. Levine (Ed.), Nebraska Symposium on Motivation (Vol. 13, pp. 123-180). University of Nebraska Press.

Premack, D., & Woodruff, G. (1978). Does the chimpanzee have a theory of mind? Behavioral and Brain Sciences, 1(4), 515-526.

Purdon, C., & Clark, D. A. (2002). The need to control thoughts. In R. O. Frost & G. Steketee (Eds.), Cognitive approaches to obsessions and compulsions: Theory, assessment, and treatment (pp. 29-43). Pergamon/Elsevier Science Inc.

Purves, D., Augustine, G. J., Fitzpatrick, D., et al. (2018). Neuroscience (6th ed.). Oxford University Press.

Puukko, K., Hietajärvi, L., Maksniemi, E., Alho, K., & Salmela-Aro, K. (2020). Social Media Use and Depressive Symptoms-A Longitudinal Study from Early to Late Adolescence. International journal of environmental research and public health, 17(16), 5921.

Qiao, H., An, S. C., Xu, C., & Ma, X. M. (2017). Role of proBDNF and BDNF in dendritic spine plasticity and depressive-like behaviors induced by an animal model of depression. Brain research, 1663, 29-37.

Qu, C., Huang, Y., Philippe, R., Cai, S., Derrington, E., Moisan, F., & Dreher, J.-C. (2023). Causal role of the medial prefrontal cortex in learning social hierarchy. bioRxiv.

Rachman S. (1997). A cognitive theory of obsessions. Behaviour research and therapy, 35(9), 793-802.

Rachman S. (2002). A cognitive theory of compulsive checking. Behaviour research and therapy, 40(6), 625-639.

Radovic, A., Gmelin, T., Stein, B. D., & Miller, E. (2017). Depressed adolescents' positive and negative use of social media. Journal of adolescence, 55, 5-15.

Rahman, S., & McBride, W. J. (2001). D1-D2 dopamine receptor interaction within the nucleus accumbens mediates long-loop negative feedback to the ventral tegmental area (VTA). Journal of neurochemistry, 77(5), 1248-1255.

Rainie, L., & Wellman, B. (2012). Networked: The new social operating system. MIT Press.

Rastogi, R. B., Lapierre, Y. D., & Singhal, R. L. (1977). Evidence for the role of brain norepinephrine and dopamine in "rebound" phenomenon seen during withdrawal after repeated exposure to benzodiazepines. Journal of psychiatric research, 13(2), 65-75.

Reijntjes, A. H. A., Thomaes, S., Boelen, P., van der Schoot, M., De Castro, B. O., Telch, M. (2011). Delighted when approved by others, to pieces when rejected: children's social anxiety magnifies the linkage between self- and otherevaluations. Journal of Child Psychology and Psychiatry, and Allied Disciplines, 52(7), 774-781.

Renfrew, C. (2007). Prehistory: The making of the human mind. Modern Library.

Rescorla, R. A., & Wagner, A. R. (1972). A Theory of Pavlovian Conditioning: Variations in the Effectiveness of Reinforcement and Nonreinforcement. Classical Conditioning II: Current Research and Theory, 64-99.

Ressler, K. J., & Nemeroff, C. B. (2000). Role of serotonergic and noradrenergic systems in the pathophysiology of depression and anxiety disorders. Depression and anxiety, 12 Suppl 1, 2-19.

Rheingold, H. (2000). The virtual community: Homesteading on the electronic frontier. MIT Press.

Richerson, P. J., & Boyd, R. (2005). Not by genes alone: How culture transformed human evolution. University of Chicago Press.

Richins, M. L. (1991). Social comparison and the idealized images of advertising. Journal of Consumer Research, 18(1), 71-83.

Roberts, S. R., & David, M. E. (2020). The social media feedback loop and self-esteem: Why we "like" social media. Computers in Human Behavior, 114, 106568.

Robinson, E. S., Dalley, J. W., Theobald, D. E., Glennon, J. C., Pezze, M. A., Murphy, E. R., & Robbins, T. W. (2008). Opposing roles for 5-HT2A and 5-HT2C receptors in the nucleus accumbens on inhibitory response control in the 5choice serial reaction time task. Neuropsychopharmacology : official publication of the American College of Neuropsychopharmacology, 33(10), 2398-2406.

Robinson, L. (2017). The identity curation game: digital inequality, identity work, and emotion management. Information, Communication & Society, 21(5), 661-680.

Rocha, B. A., Goulding, E. H., O'Dell, L. E., Mead, A. N., Coufal, N. G., Parsons, L. H., & Tecott, L. H. (2002). Enhanced locomotor, reinforcing, and neurochemical effects of cocaine in serotonin 5-hydroxytryptamine 2C receptor mutant mice. The Journal of neuroscience : the official journal of the Society for Neuroscience, 22(22), 10039-10045.

Rogers, C. R. (1951). Client-centered therapy: Its current practice, implications, and theory. Houghton Mifflin.

Rojek, C. (1995). Decentring leisure: Rethinking leisure theory. Sage Publications.

Roseboom, P. H., Coon, S. L., Baler, R., McCune, S. K., Weller, J. L., & Klein, D. C. (1996). Melatonin synthesis: analysis of the more than 150 -fold nocturnal increase in serotonin N -acetyltransferase messenger ribonucleic acid in the rat pineal gland. Endocrinology, 137(7), 3033-3045.

Rosen, J. C. (1995). The nature of body dysmorphic disorder and treatment with cognitive behavior therapy. Cognitive and Behavioral Practice, 2(1), 143-166.

Rosenthal-von der Pütten, A. M., Hastall, M. R., Köcher, S., Meske, C., Heinrich, T., Labrenz, F., & Ocklenburg, S. (2019). "Likes" as social rewards: Their role in online social comparison and decisions to like other people's selfies. Computers in Human Behavior, 92, 76-86.

Rossato, J. I., Radiske, A., Kohler, C. A., Gonzalez, C., Bevilaqua, L. R. M., Medina, J. H., & Cammarota, M. (2013). Consolidation of object recognition memory requires simultaneous activation of dopamine D1/D5 receptors in the amygdala and medial prefrontal cortex. Neurobiology of Learning and Memory, 106, 66-70.

Rubenstein J. L. (1998). Development of serotonergic neurons and their projections. Biological psychiatry, 44(3), 145-150.

Saberi, B. (2019). Reward System Components in Addictive Disorders. Open Access J Addict & Psychol, 2(2).

Sadkowski, M., Dennis, B., Clayden, R. C., Elsheikh, W., Rangarajan, S., Dejesus, J., & Samaan, Z. (2013). The role of the serotonergic system in suicidal behavior. Neuropsychiatric disease and treatment, 9, 1699-1716.

Sahlins, M. (1972). Stone age economics. Aldine de Gruyter.

Salgado-Pineda, P., Delaveau, P., Blin, O., & Nieoullon, A. (2005). Dopaminergic contribution to the regulation of emotional perception. Clinical neuropharmacology, 28(5), 228-237.

Salkovskis P. M. (1985). Obsessional-compulsive problems: a cognitive-behavioural analysis. Behaviour research and therapy, 23(5), 571-583.

Sari Y. (2004). Serotonin1B receptors: from protein to physiological function and behavior. Neuroscience and biobehavioral reviews, 28(6), 565-582.

Schudson, M. (1984). Advertising, the uneasy persuasion: Its dubious impact on American society. Basic Books.

Schultz W. (1998). Predictive reward signal of dopamine

neurons. Journal of neurophysiology, 80(1), 1-27.

Schultz W. (2006). Behavioral theories and the neuro-physiology of reward. Annual review of psychology, 57, 87-115.

Schultz W. (2007). Multiple dopamine functions at different time courses. Annual review of neuroscience, 30, 259288.

Schultz, W. (1961). Principles of operant conditioning. Journal of Experimental Psychology, 61(5), 343-353.

Schultz, W. (1998). Predictive reward signal of dopamine neurons. J Neurophysiol 80(1):1-27.

Schultz, W. (2002). Getting formal with dopamine and reward. Neuron, 36, 241-263.

Schultz, W. (2015). Neuronal reward and decision signals: From theories to data. Physiol Rev 95:853-951.

Schunk, D. H. (1987). Peer models and children's behavioral change. Review of Educational Research, 57(2), 149-174.

Schweimer, J., & Hauber, W. (2006). Dopamine D1 receptors in the anterior cingulate cortex regulate effort-based decision making. Learning & Memory, 13(6), 777-782.

Seid-Fatemi, A., & Tobler, P. N. (2015). Efficient learning mechanisms hold in the social domain and are implemented in the medial prefrontal cortex. Social Cognitive and Affective Neuroscience, 10(5), 735-742.

Seiler, J. L., Cosme, C. V., Sherathiya, V. N., Schaid, M. D., Bianco, J. M., Bridgemohan, A. S., & Lerner, T. N. (2022). Dopamine signaling in the dorsomedial striatum promotes compulsive behavior. Current biology : CB, 32(5), 1175-1188.e5.

Sennett, R. (1977). The fall of public man. Knopf.

Şentürk, E., Geniş, B., & Coşar, B. (2021). Social Media Addiction in Young Adult Patients with Anxiety Disorders and Depression. Alpha psychiatry, 22(5), 257-262.

Service, E. R. (1962). Primitive social organization: An evolutionary perspective. Random House.

Sesack, S. R., & Pickel, V. M. (1992). Prefrontal cortical efferents in the rat synapse on unlabeled neuronal targets of catecholamine terminals in the nucleus accumbens septi and on dopamine neurons in the ventral tegmental area. Journal of Comparative Neurology.

Sesack, S., & Grace, A. (2010). Cortico-basal ganglia reward network: Microcircuitry. Neuropsychopharmacology.

Shannon, H., Bush, K., Villeneuve, P. J., Hellemans, K. G., & Guimond, S. (2022). Problematic Social Media Use in Adolescents and Young Adults: Systematic Review and Meta-analysis. JMIR mental health, 9(4), e33450.

Sheng, M., & Lee, S. H. (2001). AMPA receptor trafficking and the control of synaptic transmission. Cell, 105(7), 825-828.

Sherman, L. E., Hernandez, L. M., Greenfield, P. M., & Dapretto, M. (2018). What the brain 'likes': Neural correlates of providing feedback on social media. Social Cognitive and Affective Neuroscience, 13(7), 699-707.

Sherman, L. E., Payton, A. A., Hernandez, L. M., Greenfield, P. M., & Dapretto, M. (2016). The Power of the Like in Adolescence: Effects of Peer Influence on Neural and Behavioral Responses to Social Media. Psychological science, 27(7), 1027-1035.

Shiah, I. S., & Yatham, L. N. (2000). Serotonin in mania and in the mechanism of action of mood stabilizers: a review of clinical studies. Bipolar disorders, 2(2), 77-92.

Sikora, M., et al. (2017). Ancient genomes show social and reproductive behavior of early Upper Paleolithic foragers. Science.

Simmel, G. (1971). On individuality and social forms. University of Chicago Press.

Skinner, B. F. (1938). The Behavior of Organisms: An Experimental Analysis. Appleton-Century.

Skinner, B. F. (1953). Science and Human Behavior. Macmillan.

Smith, A. (2005). The wealth of nations. (Original work published 1776). University of Chicago Press.

Smith, L. G. E., Amiot, C. E., Smith, J. R., Callan, V., Terry, D. (2013). The social validation and coping model of organizational identity development. Journal of Management, 39, 1952-1978.

Snyder, S. H., Borjigin, J., & Sassone-Corsi, P. (2006). Discovering light effects on the brain. The American journal of psychiatry, 163(5), 771.

Sokolowski, J. D., & Seiden, L. S. (1999). The behavioral effects of sertraline, fluoxetine, and paroxetine differ on the differential-reinforcement-of-low-rate 72-second operant schedule in the rat. Psychopharmacology, 147(2), 153-161.

Soubrié, P. (1986). Reconciling the role of central serotonin neurons in human and animal behavior. Behavioral and Brain Sciences, 9(2): 319-335.

Strano, D. A., & Petrocelli, J. V. (2005). A preliminary examination of the role of inferiority feelings in the academic achievement of college students. The Journal of Individual Psychology, 61(1), 81-90.

Stubbendorff, C., & Stevenson, C. W. (2021). Dopamine regulation of contextual fear and associated neural circuit function. The European journal of neuroscience, 54(8), 6933-6947.

Stuber, G. D., Klanker, M., de Ridder, B., Bowers, M. S., Joosten, R. N., Feenstra, M. G., & Bonci, A. (2008). Reward-predictive cues enhance excitatory synaptic strength onto midbrain dopamine neurons. Science (New York, N.Y.), 321(5896), 1690-1692.

Sutcliffe, A., Dunbar, R., Binder, J., & Arrow, H. (2012). Relationships and the social brain: Integrating psychological and evolutionary perspectives. British Journal of Psychology, 103(2), 149-168.

Sweeney, T. J. (1998). Adlerian counseling and psychotherapy. Accelerated Development.

Syed, E. C., Grima, L. L., Magill, P. J., Bogacz, R., Brown, P., & Walton, M. E. (2016). Action initiation shapes mesolimbic dopamine encoding of future rewards. Nature neuroscience, 19(1), 34-36.

Szewczyk, P., Szewczyk, A., & Poniewierka, E. (2018). Melatonin - Metabolism and the Role of Pineal Hormone.

Nursing and Public Health 8 (2), 135-139.

Taber, M. T., Das, S., & Fibiger, H. C. (1995). Cortical regulation of subcortical dopamine release: Mediation via the ventral tegmental area. Journal of Neurochemistry.

Tajfel, H., & Turner, J. C. (1979). An integrative theory of intergroup conflict. In W. G. Austin & S. Worchel (Eds.), The social psychology of intergroup relations (pp. 33-47). Brooks/Cole.

Takahashi J. S. (1991). Circadian rhythms: from gene expression to behavior. Current opinion in neurobiology, 1(4), 556-561.

Takahashi, H., Kato, M., Matsuura, M., Mobbs, D., Suhara, T., & Okubo, Y. (2009). When your gain is my pain and your pain is my gain: Neural correlates of envy and schadenfreude. Science, 323(5916), 937-939.

Takahashi, Y. K., Roesch, M., Wilson, R. C., Toreson, K., O'Donnell, P., Niv, Y., & Schoenbaum, G. (2011). Expectancy-related changes in firing of dopamine neurons depend on orbitofrontal cortex. Nature Neuroscience, 14, 1590-1597.

Tan, Y. T., Rehm, I. C., Stevenson, J. L., & De Foe, A. (2021). Social Media Peer Support Groups for ObsessiveCompulsive and Related Disorders: Understanding the Predictors of Negative Experiences. Journal of affective disorders, 281, 661-672.

Taylor, C. (1989). Sources of the self: The making of the modern identity. Harvard University Press.

Thierry, A., Gioanni, Y., Dégénétais, E., & Glowinski, J. (2000). Hippocampo-prefrontal cortex pathway: Anatomical and electrophysiological characteristics. Hippocampus.

Thompson, E. P. (1963). The making of the English working class. Penguin Books.

Thorisdottir, I. E., Sigurvinsdottir, R., Asgeirsdottir, B. B., Allegrante, J. P., & Sigfusdottir, I. D. (2019). Active and Passive Social Media Use and Symptoms of Anxiety and Depressed Mood Among Icelandic Adolescents. Cyberpsychology, behavior and social networking, 22(8), 535-542.

Tiggemann, M., & McGill, B. (2004). The role of social comparison in the effect of magazine advertisements on women's mood and body dissatisfaction. Journal of Social and Clinical Psychology, 23(1), 23-44.

Tiggemann, M., & Slater, A. (2013). NetGirls: The Internet, Facebook, and body image concern in adolescent girls. International Journal of Eating Disorders, 46(6), 630-633.

Titulaer, J., Björkholm, C., Feltmann, K., Malmlöf, T., Mishra, D., Bengtsson Gonzales, C., & Schilström, B. (2021). The Importance of Ventral Hippocampal Dopamine and Norepinephrine in Recognition Memory. Frontiers in Behavioral Neuroscience.

Tomasello, M. (2008). Origins of human communication. MIT Press.

Tomasello, M. (2014). A natural history of human thinking. Harvard University Press.

Traynelis, S. F., Wollmuth, L. P., McBain, C. J., Menniti, F. S., Vance, K. M., Ogden, K. K., Hansen, K. B., Yuan, H., Myers, S. J., & Dingledine, R. (2010). Glutamate receptor ion channels: structure, regulation, and function. Pharmacological reviews, 62(3), 405-496.

Triandis, H. C. (1995). Individualism & collectivism. Westview Press.

Tse, W. S., & Bond, A. J. (2002). Serotonergic intervention affects both social dominance and affiliative behaviour. Psychopharmacology, 161(3), 324-330.

Tsetsenis, T., Badyna, J. K., Wilson, J. A., Zhang, X., Krizman, E. N., Subramaniyan, M., Yang, K., Thomas, S., & Dani, J. A. (2021). Midbrain dopaminergic innervation of the hippocampus is sufficient to modulate formation of aversive memories. Proceedings of the National Academy of Sciences.

Tsetsenis, T., Broussard, J., & Dani, J. A. (2023). Dopaminergic regulation of hippocampal plasticity, learning, and memory. Frontiers in Behavioral Neuroscience.

Tükel, R., Polat, A., Ozdemir, O., Aksüt, D., & Türksoy, N. (2002). Comorbid conditions in obsessive-compulsive disorder. Comprehensive psychiatry, 43(3), 204-209.

Turchin, P. (2015). Ultrasociety: How 10,000 years of

war made humans the greatest cooperators on Earth. Beresta Books.

Turkle, S. (2011). Alone together: Why we expect more from technology and less from each other. Basic Books.

Turner, J. (1975). Social comparison and social identity: Some prospects for intergroup behaviour. European Journal of Social Psychology, 5, 1-34.

Turner, J. C. (1985). Social categorization and the self-concept: A social cognitive theory of group behavior. In E. J. Lawler (Ed.), Advances in group processes (Vol. 2, pp. 77-122). JAI Press.

Turner, J. H. (1991). The structure of sociological theory. Wadsworth Publishing.

Turner, V. (1969). The ritual process: Structure and anti-structure. Aldine de Gruyter.

Twenge, J. M. (2018). iGen: Why today's super-connected kids are growing up less rebellious, more tolerant, less happy - and completely unprepared for adulthood. Atria Books.

Vaidya, V. A., & Duman, R. S. (2001). Depresssion–emerging insights from neurobiology. British medical bulletin, 57,61-79.

Vaillant, G. E. (1993). The wisdom of the ego. Harvard University Press.

Valencia-Torres, L., Olarte-Sánchez, C. M., Lyons, D. J., Georgescu, T., Greenwald-Yarnell, M., Myers, M. G., Jr., Bradshaw, C. M., & Heisler, L. K. (2017). Activation of ventral tegmental area 5-HT2C receptors reduces incentive motivation. Neuropsychopharmacology, 42(7), 1511-1521.

Valkenburg, P. M., & Peter, J. (2011). Online communication among adolescents: an integrated model of its attraction, opportunities, and risks. The Journal of adolescent health : official publication of the Society for Adolescent Medicine, 48(2), 121-127.

Valkenburg, P. M., Peter, J., Schouten, A. P. (2006). Friend networking sites and their relationship to adolescents' well-being and social self-esteem. CyberPsychology & Behavior, 9(5), 584-590.

Van Bockstaele, E. J., Cestari, D. M., & Pickel, V. M. (1994). Synaptic structure and connectivity of serotonin terminals in the ventral tegmental area: potential sites for modulation of mesolimbic dopamine neurons. Brain research, 647(2), 307-322.

Van Dijck, J. (2013). The culture of connectivity: A critical history of social media. Oxford University Press.

Veblen, T. (1899). The theory of the leisure class: An economic study of institutions. Macmillan.

Viswanath, B., Narayanaswamy, J. C., Rajkumar, R. P., Cherian, A. V., Kandavel, T., Math, S. B., & Reddy, Y. C. (2012). Impact of depressive and anxiety disorder comorbidity on the clinical expression of obsessive-compulsive disorder. Comprehensive psychiatry, 53(6), 775-782.

Vogel, E. A., Rose, J. P., Okdie, B. M., Eckles, K., & Franz, B. (2014). Who compares and despairs? The effect of social comparison orientation on social media use and its outcomes. Personality and Individual Differences, 86, 249-256.

Vogel, E. A., Rose, J. P., Roberts, L. R., & Eckles, K. (2014). Social comparison, social media, and self-esteem. Psychology of Popular Media Culture, 3(4), 206-222.

Volkow, N. D., Fowler, J. S., Wang, G. J., & Goldstein, R. Z. (2002). Role of dopamine, the frontal cortex and memory circuits in drug addiction: insight from imaging studies. Neurobiology of learning and memory, 78(3), 610624 .

Volkow, N. D., Fowler, J. S., Wang, G. J., Baler, R., & Telang, F. (2009). Imaging dopamine's role in drug abuse and addiction. Neuropharmacology, 56 Suppl 1(Suppl 1), 3-8.

Volkow, N. D., Fowler, J. S., Wang, G. J., Swanson, J. M., & Telang, F. (2007). Dopamine in drug abuse and addiction: results of imaging studies and treatment implications. Archives of neurology, 64(11), 1575-1579.

Volkow, N. D., Wang, G. J., Fowler, J. S., Tomasi, D., & Telang, F. (2011). Addiction: beyond dopamine reward circuitry. Proceedings of the National Academy of Sciences of the United States of America, 108(37), 15037-15042.

Volkow, N. D., Wise, R. A., & Baler, R. (2017). The dopamine motive system: implications for drug and food addiction. Nature reviews. Neuroscience, 18(12), 741-752.

Vollrath, L., Huesgen, A., & Pollow, K. (1988). Day/Night Serotonin Levels in the Pineal Gland of Male BALB/c Mice With Melatonin Deficiency. Acta Endocrinologica, 117 (1), 93-98.

Volz, K. G., Kessler, T., & von Cramon, D. Y. (2009). In-group as part of the self: In-group favoritism is mediated by medial prefrontal cortex activation. Social neuroscience, 4(3), 244-260.

Voon, V., Pessiglione, M., Brezing, C., Gallea, C., Fernandez, H. H., Dolan, R. J., & Hallett, M. (2010). Mechanisms underlying dopamine-mediated reward bias in compulsive behaviors. Neuron, 65(1), 135-142.

Vygotsky, L. S. (1978). Mind in society: The development of higher psychological processes. Harvard University Press.

Wadsley, M., Covey, J., & Ihssen, N. (2022). The Predictive Utility of Reward-Based Motives Underlying Excessive and Problematic Social Networking Site Use. Psychological reports, 125(5), 2485-2516.

Walther, J. B., Van Der Heide, B., Kim, S. Y., Westerman, D., & Tong, S. T. (2008). The role of friends' appearance and behavior on evaluations of individuals on Facebook: Are we known by the company we keep?. Human Communication Research, 34(1), 28-49.

Watts, R. E. (2013). Adlerian counseling. In B. J. Irby, G. Brown, R. Lara-Alecio, & S. Jackson (Eds.), The handbook of educational theories (pp. 459-472).

Whiten, A., & Byrne, R. W. (1997). Machiavellian intelligence II: Extensions and evaluations. Cambridge University Press.

Wiessner, P. (2002). Hunting, healing, and hxaro exchange: A long-term perspective on !Kung (Ju/'hoansi) large-game hunting. Evolution and Human Behavior, 23(6), 407-436.

Williams, R. (1980). Advertising: The magic system. In

Problems in materialism and culture. Verso.

Wills, T. A. (1981). Downward comparison principles in social psychology. Psychological Bulletin, 90(2), 245-271.

Wilson, A. E., & Ross, M. (2000). The frequency of temporal-self and social comparisons in people's personal appraisals. Journal of Personality and Social Psychology, 78(5), 928-942.

Wilson, R. C., Takahashi, Y. K., Schoenbaum, G., & Niv, Y. (2014). Orbitofrontal Cortex as a Cognitive Map of Task Space. Neuron, 81, 267-279.

Winstanley, C. A., Theobald, D. E., Dalley, J. W., Cardinal, R. N., & Robbins, T. W. (2006). Double dissociation between serotonergic and dopaminergic modulation of medial prefrontal and orbitofrontal cortex during a test of impulsive choice. Cerebral cortex (New York, N.Y. : 1991), 16(1), 106-114.

Winstanley, C. A., Theobald, D. E., Dalley, J. W., Glennon, J. C., & Robbins, T. W. (2004). 5-HT2A and 5-HT2C receptor antagonists have opposing effects on a measure of impulsivity: interactions with global 5-HT depletion. Psychopharmacology, 176(3-4), 376-385.

Winterer, J., Stempel, A. V., Dugladze, T., Földy, C., Maziashvili, N., Zivkovic, A. R., Priller, J., Soltesz, I., Gloveli, T., & Schmitz, D. (2011). Cell-type-specific modulation of feedback inhibition by serotonin in the hippocampus. The Journal of neuroscience : the official journal of the Society for Neuroscience, 31(23), 8464-8475.

Wood, J. V. (1989). Theory and research concerning social comparisons of personal attributes. Psychological Bulletin, 106(2), 231-248.

Woodburn, J. (1982). Egalitarian societies. Man, 17(3), 431-451.

Worsley, J. D., Mansfield, R., & Corcoran, R. (2018). Attachment Anxiety and Problematic Social Media Use: The Mediating Role of Well-Being. Cyberpsychology, behavior and social networking, 21(9), 563-568.

Xia, Y., Driscoll, J. R., Wilbrecht, L., et al. (2011). Nucleus accumbens medium spiny neurons target nondopaminergic neurons in the ventral tegmental area. The Journal of Neuroscience.

Xue, W., Wang, P., Li, B., Li, Y., Xu, X., Yang, F., Yao, X., Chen, Y. Z., Xu, F., & Zhu, F. (2016). Identification of the inhibitory mechanism of FDA approved selective serotonin reuptake inhibitors: an insight from molecular dynamics simulation study. Physical chemistry chemical physics : PCCP, 18(4), 3260-3271.

Yalçın, B., Pomrenze, M. B., Malacon, K., Drexler, R., Rogers, A. E., Shamardani, K., Chau, I. J., Taylor, K. R., Ni, L., Contreras-Esquivel, D., Malenka, R. C., & Monje, M. (2024). Myelin plasticity in the ventral tegmental area is required for opioid reward. Nature, 630(8017), 677-685.

Yang, C.-C., & Brown, B. B. (2016). Online self-presentation on Facebook and self-development during the college transition. Journal of Youth and Adolescence, 45(2), 402-416.

Yoshimoto, K., Kaneda, S., Kawai, Y., Ueda, S., Takeuchi, Y., Matsushita, H., Yuri, K., & Yasuhara, M. (1999). Treating neonatal rats with 6 -hydroxydopamine induced an increase in voluntary alcohol consumption. Alcoholism, clinical and experimental research, 23(4 Suppl), 2S-6S.

Zeiler M. D. (1968). Fixed and variable schedules of response-independent reinforcement. Journal of the experimental analysis of behavior, 11(4), 405-414.

Zhang, M., Ouagazzal, AM., Sun, BC., Creese, I. (1997). Regulation of Motor Behavior by Dopamine Receptor Subtypes. In: Neve, K.A., Neve, R.L. (Eds.). The Dopamine Receptors. The Receptors. Humana Press.

Zhao, Y., Paul, R., Reid, S. D., Vieira, C. C., Wolfe, C., Zhang, Y., & Chunara, R. (2024). Constructing social vulnerability indexes with increased data and machine learning highlight the importance of wealth across global contexts. Social Indicators Research.

Zheng, H., Patterson, L. M., & Berthoud, H. R. (2007). Food reward: Orexin-signaling in ventral tegmental area contributes to high-fat intake induced by accumbens opioid stimulation. Appetite.

Zhong, P., Yuen, E. Y., & Yan, Z. (2008). Modulation of neuronal excitability by serotonin-NMDA interactions in prefrontal cortex. Molecular and cellular neurosciences, 38(2), 290-299.

Zhou, K., Xu, H., Lu, S., Jiang, S., Hou, G., Deng, X., He, M., & Zhu, Y. (2022). Reward and aversion processing by input-defined parallel nucleus accumbens circuits in mice. Nature communications, 13(1), 6244.

About the Author

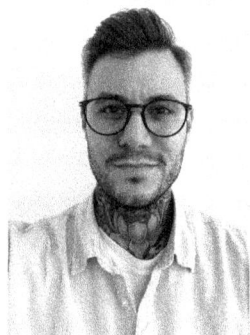

Prof. Dr. Tobey Gross is the scientific director of the Zentrum für Medienpsychologie und Verhaltenswissenschaft (ZeMV) and frequently collaborates with other scientists in an effort to understand and inform about the health implications of digital media in our modern world. He teaches psychology students in differential and personality psychology and a range of other sociology- and psychology-based disciplines, including communication. As a consultant in psychological and social professional rehabilitation, he has experience with individuals suffering from diverse mental health challenges. As the chair of the International Council of Academics for Progressive Education (I.C.A.P.E.), he is actively involved in driving science-based changes in educational environments and establishing networks among educators across the globe.

Tobey Gross is a depression patient and continually works on his own mental health.